If you have a home computer with internet access you may:
- request an item be placed on hold
- renew an item that is overdue
- view titles and due dates checked out on your card
- view your own outstanding fines

To view your patron record from your home computer:
Click on the NSPL homepage:
http://nspl.suffolk.lib.ny.us

North Shore Public Library

watch me...

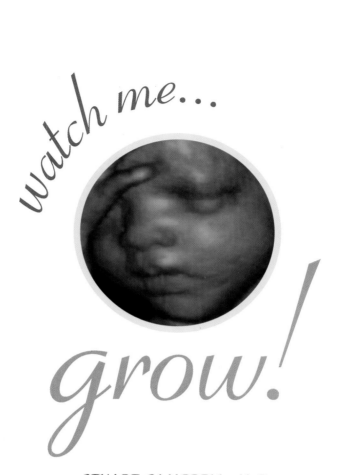

grow!

STUART CAMPBELL, M.D.

A unique, 3-DIMENSIONAL, week-by-week look at
baby's behavior and development in the womb

St. Martin's Press
New York

To my wife, Jane, and our children:
Bruce, Tiffany, Oliver, and Charles

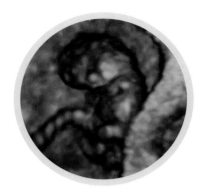

Text and illustrations © Stuart Campbell M.D. 2004
Compilation © Carroll & Brown Limited 2004

ISBN 0-312-33214-9
EAN 978-0312-33214-3
First U.S. Edition: October 2004
10 9 8 7 6 5 4 3 2 1

First published in 2004 in the United Kingdom by
Carroll & Brown Publishers Limited

Design by Emily Cook

Reproduced by Colourscan
Printed and bound in Barcelona by Book Print

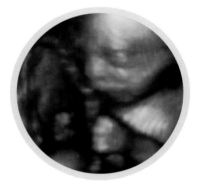

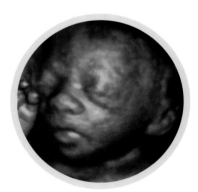

CONTENTS

There are many books for prospective parents-to-be on how they should prepare for the birth of their baby and cope with the wonderful, but in some ways strange, noisy and almost frightening newcomer in their lives. Very few of these books address in any detail the life of the baby before birth, and when they do, it is often with a mixture of inspired guesswork and a touch of fantasy. This is not surprising for until the advent of the ultrasound scan, the womb contained a private fetal world that revealed very few secrets. And even the speckled black-and-white images of the conventional 2-D ultrasound scan, which are excellent for measuring the fetus and diagnosing abnormalities, convey very little information about the behavior and emotions of the baby during its long 38-week journey from conception to birth.

But now we have a means of entering this prenatal, fetal world with a new ultrasound technique called 3-D scanning. It uses the same ultrasound waves as the conventional scan, which are known to be safe in pregnancy, but it collects the reflected sound waves not in thin slices that are difficult for non-experts to interpret, but in volumes which can be displayed in three dimensions. The resulting images provide a lifelike representation of the surface features of the baby. Even more exciting is that because the image can be updated three or four times each second (called 4-D), the movements, facial expressions, and moods of the baby can be clearly demonstrated to mother, father, relatives, and friends. This in itself has brought about a revolution. With a conventional scan, parents have to wait for the doctor or sonographer to interpret the image and point out anatomical features for them on the screen; with 3-D and 4-D scanning, they can interpret the image at the same time as the person performing the scan. This leads to a spontaneous dialogue, which I personally find very satisfying. Indeed, the first time that I saw convincing evidence of a fetus opening its eyelids was when a father exclaimed, "Look! He's opening his eyes." I was preparing to explain that as it was dark inside the uterus, this was unlikely when I realized he was right!

It has for many years been recognized that prenatal bonding between a mother and her unborn child is hugely beneficial for the emotional and even physical wellbeing of both the child and the mother herself. Many years ago, my colleagues and I showed that the conventional 2-D scan was helpful in promoting bonding before birth but now, with the experience that I have gained over the years, I can say confidently that 3-D and 4-D is much superior in this regard. The reaction of

parents to "seeing" their, as yet, unborn baby is extraordinary. The father, who frequently is a passive observer during a conventional scan, is now totally involved in the whole process. I have seen fathers kiss the screen or their partners' abdomens in an ecstasy of recognition and love for the new baby. In an age when we acknowledge that every unborn baby's life is precious, the role of this ultrasound technique in promoting bonding is indeed a new factor of great importance.

This book catalogs and describes the development and behavior of the fetus throughout pregnancy through the "window" of 3-D and 4-D ultrasound imaging. At the moment, few couples will have the opportunity to see their babies with this new technique but with the help of these images, I hope this book will enhance their understanding of the life of their babies before birth.

TWO-DIMENSIONAL ULTRASOUND

All couples will be offered 2-D ultrasound scans and, hopefully, a Doppler (see page 8) as part of their antenatal care. These scans will give their caregivers key information about the pregnancy, which will allow them to optimize antenatal care and provide each couple with information about the health of their baby.

12 Weeks Scan

Sometimes called the "first trimester scan" this is performed between 11 and 14 weeks for the following reasons:

Establish an accurate estimated delivery date Although the first day of the last menstrual period (LMP) is a guide to the age of the fetus, in about 15 percent of cases it is inaccurate in indicating when conception occurred. Measurement of the fetal crown-to-rump length, especially if performed around the end of the first trimester, is more accurate than the LMP and there is a growing consensus that the predictions made from early ultrasound measurements should be used to date all

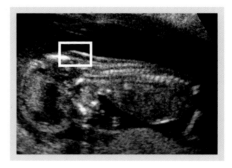

NUCHAL TRANSLUCENCY
There is an area behind the baby's neck (boxed), which contains some fluid. Ultrasound is used to measure this space and a computer program gives each mother an individualized risk for Down's syndrome based on her age and the size of the nuchal translucency.

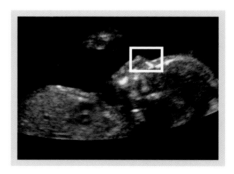

NASAL BONE LENGTH
This has recently proven to be an early and good marker for assessing the risk of Down's syndrome. In scans taken during the first trimester, if a nose bone is present the risk of Down's syndrome is reduced by a factor of three.

pregnancies. It is important to know the age of the fetus as precisely as possible especially if an intervention is subsequently needed, so that it can be carried out at the correct time. Moreover, many blood tests depend on an accurate knowledge of the dates.

Diagnose multiple gestation Twins occur in approximately 1 in 50 pregnancies. Two-thirds of these are non-identical and one-third identical. Identical twins, which are monochorionic (where the babies share a placenta), have a greater chance of complications (see page 21). For this reason, early diagnosis and monitoring are required.

Identify an increased risk for chromosome abnormalities (e.g. Down's Syndrome) Although ultrasound cannot make a precise diagnosis, certain markers will predict an increased risk. The presence of a small nuchal translucency and a nose bone are reassuring features.

20 Weeks Scan

Also called the "second trimester scan," this is performed between 18 and 22 weeks for the following reasons:

Make a detailed anatomical survey Every organ in the fetal body will be looked at to ascertain in-depth structural information. In particular the following will be examined: The skull, brain (including cerebral ventricles and cerebellum), face, spine, heart (four-chamber view and large arteries), liver, kidneys, bladder, limbs (six leg-bones and six arm-bones), feet, and hands. The doctor or sonographer will discuss these findings as the scan is performed so that you are fully informed and see the anatomy for yourself.

Placental site Sometimes the placenta lies low in the uterus and occasionally this will become *placenta previa* (i.e. lying close to or covering the cervix). This condition is associated with bleeding in the third trimester and premature birth and the obstetrician will usually decide to perform a cesarean section. Early knowledge will optimize management and secure a safe outcome.

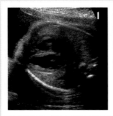

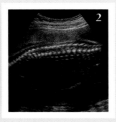

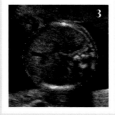

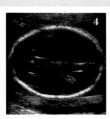

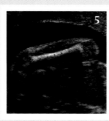

Fetal growth Measurements of your baby's head circumference (HC) and biparietal diameter (BPD), abdominal circumference (AC), and femur or thigh bone length (FL) will be taken to provide baseline measurements to check baby's subsequent growth.

Measurement of the cervix If the mother is at a high risk of having a premature birth (e.g. previous early delivery or twins), then a cervical measurement is helpful in prediciting the likelihood of premature labor. A cervical length of less than half an inch (1.5cm) indicates a high risk.

Doppler Ultrasound

Advanced ultrasound departments now offer an assessment of uterine artery flow. This is important in first pregnancies. The two uterine arteries on each side of the uterus are mapped out in color by Doppler and the flow waveforms from these arteries are analyzed. If there is good flow on the beginning (systole) and end (diastole) of the waveform, the growth of the baby should be normal. If the waveform has a notch with poor flow in diastole, then there is a risk of slow growth of the fetus and high blood pressure (pre-eclampsia) in the mother.

ASSESSMENTS AT 20 WEEKS
During this scan, the sonographer will want to check on all the organs of the body and take some useful measurements.

When the heart is visualized (1), the sonographer will check to see that it is occupying about a third of the chest and points to the left; that there are four chambers, which are equal in size; and that the major arteries are connected correctly.

The spine (2) will be examined to ensure that the posterior spinous process is present along its length in order to rule out neural tube defects.

Baseline measurements will be taken of the abdominal circumference (3) head circumference (4), and the length of a femur, one of the leg bones (5).

Further Ultrasounds

These can be carried out at any time in the following cases:

- You're carrying twins or more babies
- Your doctor suspects your baby is too small or too large for its age
- You have too little or too much amniotic fluid
- You're at risk for premature labor
- You have diabetes, hypertension, or other underlying medical condition
- You're bleeding

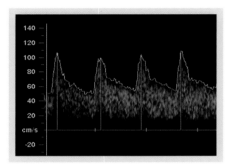

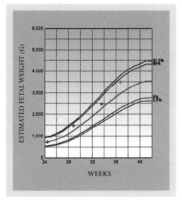

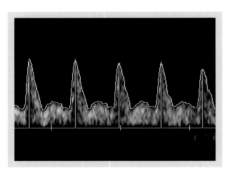

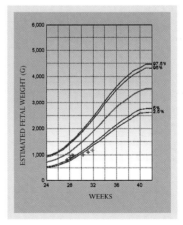

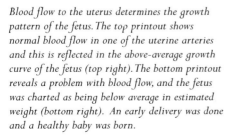

Blood flow to the uterus determines the growth pattern of the fetus. The top printout shows normal blood flow in one of the uterine arteries and this is reflected in the above-average growth curve of the fetus (top right). The bottom printout reveals a problem with blood flow, and the fetus was charted as being below average in estimated weight (bottom right). An early delivery was done and a healthy baby was born.

A Word About Dates

Pregnancy is conventionally divided into three time periods called trimesters. This is inconvenient for, however you calculate the duration of pregnancy, the number of weeks is not divisible by three. Convention also dictates that the duration of pregnancy is calculated from the first day of the mother's last menstrual period (LMP), and so a "typical" pregnancy lasts 40 weeks (though gestation, the actual age of the fetus, is regarded as being two weeks less). This also is confusing because if a woman's periods are irregular, this date is clearly not an accurate guide to the age of the fetus. From my perspective, however, it makes sense that there are two short trimesters of 12 weeks each and a longer one of 16 weeks. This is because the three trimesters demarcate distinct phases in fetal development.

In the first trimester (weeks 1-12), the baby's organs develop and should be complete by the end of this time.

In the second trimester (weeks 13-24) the baby's growth is rapid and he or she develops the ability to perform complex coordinated activities. By the end of this period the baby is regarded as viable, i.e. capable of surviving outside the womb, albeit with the expert assistance of a pediatric team.

In the third trimester (weeks 25-40), the baby puts on weight and develops behavioral patterns, which prepare him or her for life outside the womb.

Trimester 1

During the first trimester (weeks 1-12), the fetus develops from a single fertilized egg into a complete, and very complex, organism. This is a period of frantic development: cells multiply, migrate, and re-group; forming layers of tissues that fold and unfold. In just three to six weeks, a basic body plan is laid down.

7 WEEKS PREGNANCY

Once the initial ball of cells implants in the uterine wall, a remarkable chain of events is set into motion. The embryo's three germ-layers begin to differentiate into specialized cells that are critical for life such as blood cells, nerve cells, and kidney cells.

10 WEEKS PREGNANCY

Overall growth is fast and highly coordinated. External features such as the face, eyes, ear, arms, and legs appear first. Internally, the heart is one of the first organs to be recognized. It starts beating at about the 22nd day following fertilization. The brain and spinal cord, and the respiratory, gastrointestinal, and genitourinary systems start to develop simultaneously.

The musculoskeletal system will start developing during the second half of the first trimester. By ten weeks (eight weeks gestation), the developing baby is known as a fetus, and contains all the organs and structures found in a full-term newborn but in an immature state.

The baby's life support system, in the form of the umbilical cord and placenta, develops simultaneously. Initially, the baby develops within its amniotic sac, which is contained within the chorionic sac, but by the end of this trimester these two have fused together.

The first trimester is, however, the period when the developing baby is most at risk from genetic problems and from external sources such as infection, radiation, nutritional imbalances, and teratogens (birth-defect causing factors). Therefore, it's not surprising that most miscarriages happen at this time, including many where the mother is unaware that she is pregnant.

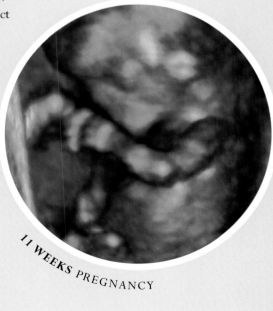

11 WEEKS PREGNANCY

Weeks 1-5

Conception begins when a sperm fertilizes an egg and a zygote is formed. Over the next few days, the zygote divides rapidly while it makes its way down the fallopian tube into the uterus. There it implants and splits into two sets of cells; about half will become the placenta and the other half will become the fetus.

By the second week after conception, your baby has developed from a hollow ball of cells (blastocyst) into a flat disc shape (embryonic disc). The three germ-layers from which all your baby's organs will develop appear now. These are the ectoderm (skin, nerve tissue), endoderm (liver, intestines), and mesoderm (bone, muscles).

During the third week after conception, the embryonic disc folds into a cylinder as it develops a head and tail. By day 22, a primitive heart, shaped as a tube in a loop, begins to beat. Thus, very primitive blood cells start to circulate through forming minute blood vessels. The early beginnings of the nervous system appear when a sheet of cells on the embryo's back folds in the middle and by day 28, form a tube (neural tube) that will become the spinal cord. After this the head of the embryo begins to grow rapidly and within it the upper part of the neural tube expands to form the brain. At the top early signs of eyes and ears emerge.

Your baby also has a support system, in the form of a yolk sac which, connected to the embryo's developing gut system by the vitelline duct, operates as an exchange organ for nutrients and disposal of waste to and from the embryo. The yolk sac supports the growth of the embryo until the placenta gradually takes over between weeks 8 and 9, which is a critical time in the embryo's development.

Week

From the sixth week of pregnancy, my growth is very rapid. Though my heart is only as big as a poppy seed, and only has one chamber, it's beginning to beat on its own and blood has started to circulate through my tiny blood vessels.

My neural tube will close and my digestive tract begins to form; I have a foregut, midgut, and hindgut. Present in very primitive form are my lungs, liver, pancreas, and thyroid.

Facial features are starting to form; my nostrils are becoming distinct. My neck and jaw start to develop. I've assumed a distinctive C-shape and my head and tail ends are easily discernible. Tiny buds, which will turn into my arms and legs, have begun to appear.

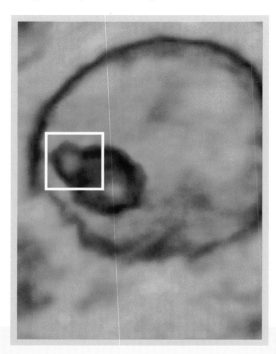

GESTATION
4 weeks

LENGTH
½₂ to ⅙ inch (2 to 4 mm)
from crown to rump

You can see a 4-week-old embryo (boxed) attached to his yolk sac; both are contained within the chorionic sac. At this stage of development the placenta has not yet formed properly, so the yolk sac has a very important role. It passes essential nutrients via a membrane to the early embryo.

Week 7

GESTATION
5 weeks

LENGTH
⅙ to ⅕ inch (4 to 5 mm)
from crown to rump

I've grown to look like a small bean with a bumpy head that bends forward and is proportionally much larger than the rest of my body. My back is gently curved and my tail is gradually disappearing. There are dark spots on the sides of my head, which are my eyes forming. Little openings on my face mark my nostrils and on either side of my neck, my ears are developing.

My arm- and leg-buds protrude more, the beginnings of my elbows

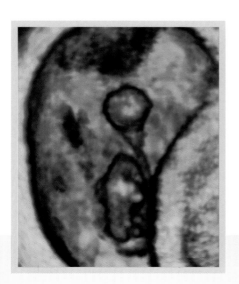

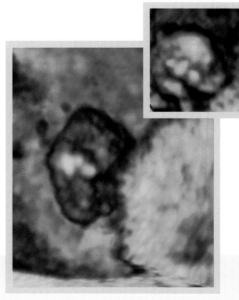

appear, and my hands and feet are paddle-shaped. My foot length is a tiny fraction of an inch.

Internally, my brain has divided into distinct segments and my cerebral hemispheres are growing fast as are my muscle fibers. Within a few days these will begin to move for the first time. My heart, which bulges out, is becoming a four-chambered organ, and is beating about 150 beats a minute — twice my mother's rate! Main air passageways or bronchi are forming in my lungs.

My intestines are developing and my appendix and pancreas are present. Part of my intestines bulge into the umbilical cord. My internal sex organs are now nearing completion.

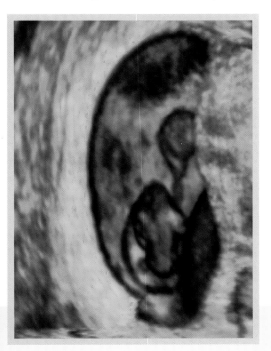

The embryo has grown considerably and is now larger than his yolk sac. The latter is joined to the embryo's gut and blood vessels and continues to provide nourishment as the placental circulation is not yet properly established.

The embryo has two distinct ends — head and tail — and limb buds are apparent. The inset picture gives a good view of phangeal arches: These are the structures from which the face will develop.

The embryo sits in a sac within a sac. Visible in the last picture is the outline of the amniotic sac, which is found within the larger chorionic (placental) sac. By the beginning of the second trimester, the amniotic sac will completely fill the chorionic sac and the two will fuse to form the gestational sac.

Week

GESTATION
6 weeks

LENGTH
½ to ¾ inch (14 to 20 mm)
from crown to rump

My head is still the largest part of my body and remains bent forward on my chest. However, my trunk is longer in proportion to my head and I'm less of a C-shape.

My facial features continue to develop. I have a rudimentary nose with nostrils, and my jaw is fusing to shape my mouth in which I have a tongue. My eyes are open and positioned very widely apart (about 160°), so that they seem to be on the sides of my head rather than in front. My eyelids are just

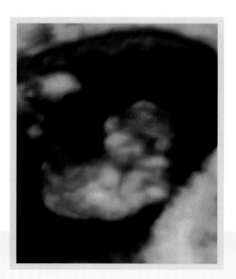

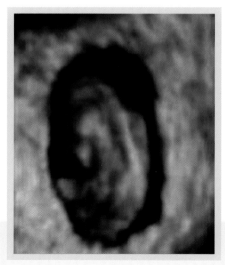

WEEK 8

discernible and my inner, but not outer, ear is developing.

Most of my internal organs – heart, brain, liver, lungs, and kidneys – have developed in a basic form and my intestines are so long they have to continue their development outside the abdomen, within a sac adjacent to the umbilical cord.

My arms and legs are longer and project straight forward and my hands can bend at the wrist.

Crown-to-rump measurements

During ultrasound examinations, a measurement is taken from the top of a baby's head (crown) to his bottom (rump). This is considered the most accurate method for determining fetal age in pregnancy and can be obtained as early as seven weeks. This accuracy is possible because fetuses follow a very predictable growth rate in the first trimester. When your baby's measurement is compared to a set of standard lengths, the result is an estimated age that is considered to be accurate within five days.

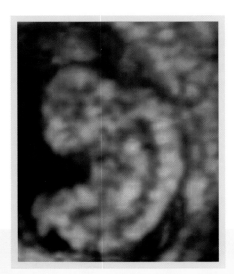

At this stage you can notice several features. The first two pictures show the outer surface of the baby's body and are "external scans" of the side and back surface of the baby, while the third picture reveals inner structures.

In the central picture, you can make out an arm- and a leg-bud and the spinal column. In the last picture, you can see clearly inside the baby and make out the individual vertebral bodies of the backbone.

The yolk sac now is tiny compared to the embryo and you can see the umbilical cord leading from the placenta to the umbilicus.

Week 9

GESTATION
7 weeks

LENGTH
1 inch (22 to 30 mm) from
crown to rump

I think I'm beginning to look more like a baby! My back is less curved and my neck is forming while my "tail" has disappeared. My arms and legs are much longer and growing fast. My fingers and toes are almost complete – and I have touch pads on my fingers.

My eyelids almost cover my eyes, my jaw is completely formed, and I have a nose.

My intestines are moving back into my abdominal cavity, which is now getting big enough to house them.

Both knee and elbow joints now are visible and the embryo is capable of some movement. See if you can spot the difference in leg position between the two pictures, right. The swollen umbilical cord contains the developing intestines. These will soon move back to the abdominal cavity.

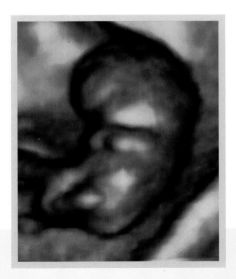

Mono- and Di-chorionic Twins

When a single fertilized egg divides, identical twins are the result, most of which are monochorionic. Two eggs, fertilized at the same time, produce fraternal or di-chorionic twins (each having his own chorionic sac). Monochorionic twins have one placenta and lie in one chorionic sac, although in many cases they are surrounded by their own amniotic sacs. Monochorionic twin pregnancies have more complications than dichorionic because sometimes one twin will leak blood into the circulation of the other (called twin-twin transfusion syndrome). In most cases, if spotted early, the condition can be treated successfully.

Sometimes laser surgery is used on the placenta to "stop the leak." This is why your obstetrician will want to know as early as possible if you are carrying twins, and what kind of twins they are. This scan shows a mono-dichorionic triplet pregnancy – monochorionic twins and a singleton sibling in his own placental sac.

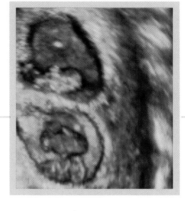

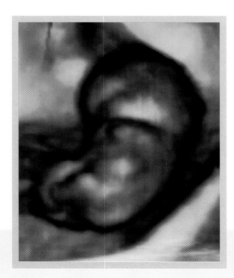

Week 10

GESTATION
8 weeks

LENGTH
1¼ to 1⅔ inches (31 to 42 mm) from crown to rump

WEIGHT
⅕ ounce (5 g)

At this week I'm officially known as a fetus, which means "offspring." Before this time, my weight was too little to calculate but now it can be measured to show weekly differences.

My brain has grown a lot, so that my head still looks very big in proportion to the rest of my body. My eyes and nose are clearly visible, but my eyelids are fused and won't open until after the

Compare this fetus with the one at 9 weeks and you'll see how much progress there can be in a week. At this stage, all babies are much the same size so doctors are able to date gestation from scans quite accurately.

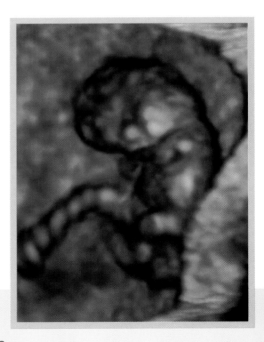

24 weeks (but see week 18). Twenty tiny tooth buds (baby teeth) are forming in my gums.

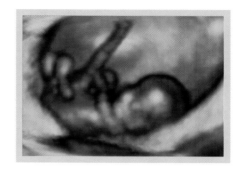

Most of my joints have formed, including my wrists and ankles. My fingers and toes are visible and separated, and my foot is approximately 1/10th of an inch.

My nervous system is responsive and many of my internal organs have begun to function. My heart has attained its final shape; it now beats at 140 beats per minute. My lungs continue to develop, as do my stomach and my intestines. My kidneys are moving into their final positions in my upper abdomen.

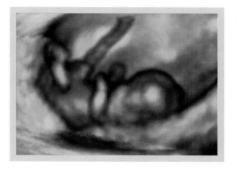

It's much easier to see limb movement in a fetus of 8 weeks' gestation than in one of 7 weeks' gestation. In the bottom picture, the baby is holding his hands in the commonly observed "boxer" position. The bulge in the umbilical cord is the fetus' developing intestines.

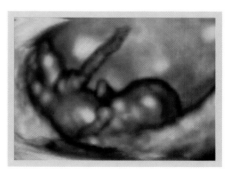

Week 11

GESTATION
9 weeks

LENGTH
1¼ to 2¼ inches (44 to 60 mm) from crown to rump

WEIGHT
⅓ ounce (8 g)

All my vital organs – brain, lungs, liver, kidneys, and intestines – are fully formed and are increasing in volume. By the end of this week, I'll have practically doubled my body length since last week but my head is about half the length.

In my eyes, the irises are starting to develop and by the end of the week my ear's internal development will be complete.

On a scan, my fingers can now be counted and I can swallow, yawn, and suck.

The two scans shown here were taken from different positions. The one on the left is a trans-abdominal scan while the one on the right was taken vaginally. You can see that the eyes have moved more to the center of the face and that the eyelids are present. The ears are starting to assume their final shape. Now, there are no intestines in the base of the cord.

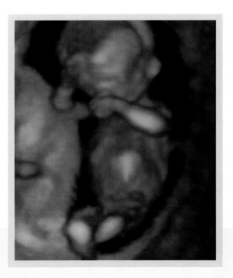

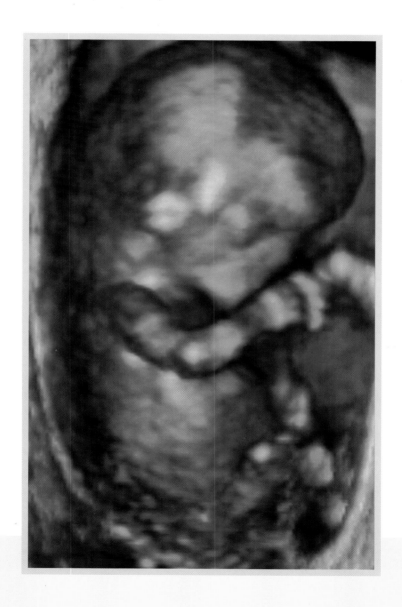

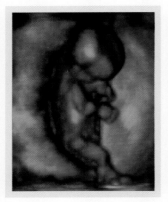 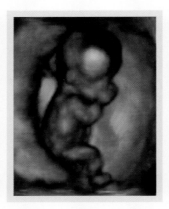 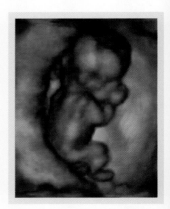

During the latter part of the first trimester, the baby moves his head and limbs but on the cusp of entering the second trimester he starts leaping, using the walls of the uterus as a springboard.

In this sequence, the fetus exhibits behavior identical to what he will do after birth, if he's held upright on a flat surface – he'll try and move forward; this is known as the walking or the stepping reflex.

This is one of the earliest seen examples of reflex behavior, and reflexes in general begin developing early. They are essential to a baby's survival so he is given plenty of time to perfect them.

In his fluid-filled amniotic sac, this baby brings his leg up, bends his knee at the joint, then carefully places his foot flat down on the uterine surface. These are commonly observed phenomena along with the

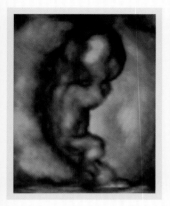 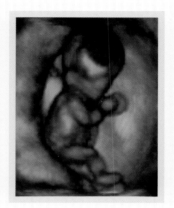 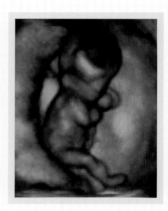

position of his hands. They are either held to his mouth or in front of his face in what's known as the boxing position. He has a limited number of weeks in which there's the space to move so freely and he's making the most of it.

The skull bones in his head are widely separated; this ensures that his brain is able to develop unimpeded.

"Were it ever so airy a tread,
My heart would hear her and beat"

Week 12

GESTATION
10 weeks

LENGTH
2½ inches (61 mm) from
crown to rump

WEIGHT
⅓ to ½ ounce (8 to 14 g)

Although my organs, particularly my brain, will continue to develop, I've acquired all the individual features that make me a human being. Also, I've almost doubled in size over the past three weeks!

My fingers and toes have separated, my hair and nails continue to grow, and my bones are hardening due to the laying down of calcium.

My genital organs are clearly discernible (look at the middle picture) although only an expert could say

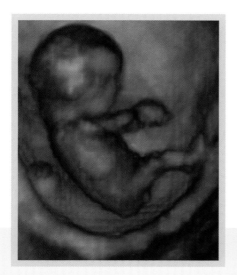

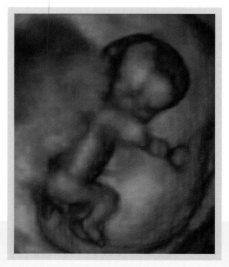

whether I am a boy or girl. What you can't see is that my vocal cords are forming and my pituitary gland, at the base of my brain, is beginning to make hormones.

My digestive system is now capable of producing the contractions that push food through my bowels and it can absorb glucose or sugar.

Things are really moving now, including me. I have a lot of fun stretching my arms and legs and jumping about.

Chorion Villus Sampling (CVS)

The placenta contains chorionic villi, which are tiny, finger-like pieces of tissue that have the same chromosomes and genetic make-up as the fetus. Using ultrasound as a guide, a physician can aspirate some of these cells into a needle. The cells will be examined for chromosomal abnormalities. This procedure is carried out earlier than amniocentesis (see page 41) but has a slightly higher risk of miscarriage. This increased risk is not to do with the procedure itself but because the overall rate of miscarriage is higher at 12 weeks' pregnancy than at 16 weeks.

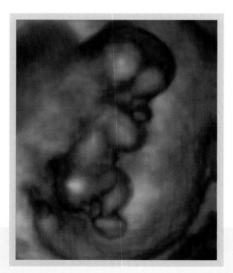

This baby is making the most of her buoyant environment, exercising her arms and legs with a range of movements that are fluid and supple. Her arms move in and out and her legs kick up and down. Her anterior fontanel (called the soft spot on a newborn) is very large; this allows her brain plenty of growing room. The placenta appears as a fluffy cloud in the last two pictures.

Trimester 2

During the second trimester (weeks 13-24), the baby's growth is rapid and he develops complex coordinated activities. Whereas in the first trimester the emphasis was on cell differentiation and then cell division (hyperplasia), now it depends solely on cell division.

13 WEEKS PREGNANCY

This is the time of the fetus' greatest activity. He can bend, stretch, kick, leap, flex, twist, and can make very complex movements with his hands. He exhibits a variety of other behavior including sucking, swallowing, yawning, spatial awareness, and grasping. There is rapid growth of your baby's cerebellum and this is responsible for his being able to develop more coordinated activities. About midway into this period, you will begin to feel your baby's movements.

17 WEEKS PREGNANCY

Nails, skin, and body hair, including eyebrows and eyelashes, appear and protective coatings of skin and nerves are produced. Ova or sperm are present.

Your baby is now capable of creating bile and urine and can hear noises; some scientists claim he can distinguish different tastes.

All his internal body systems continue to mature: including the circulatory, sensory, and hormonal, though they are not very efficient. There is a large gain in weight and length towards the end of this period.

Your baby has passed a crucial stage in his development and there is now less risk of his being affected by most infections and certain drugs, as well as developing congenital abnormalities. By the end of this period the baby is regarded as viable, i.e. capable of surviving outside the womb, albeit with the expert assistance of a pediatric team.

Antenatal tests at this time can detect birth defects and a child's gender.

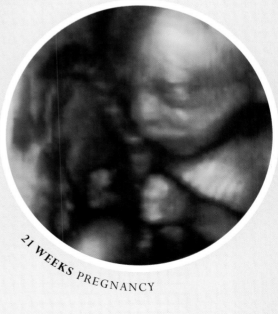

21 WEEKS PREGNANCY

Week

GESTATION
11 weeks

LENGTH
3 inches (75 mm) from
crown to rump

WEIGHT
⅔ ounce (20 g)

If my mother prods her abdomen, I will squirm. In fact, because I've acquired several reflexes: If my palms are touched, I will close my fingers; if the soles of my feet are stimulated, my toes will curl down, and if my eyelids are touched, my eye muscles will tighten.

My nerve cells have been multiplying rapidly, and synapses (neurological connections) are forming.

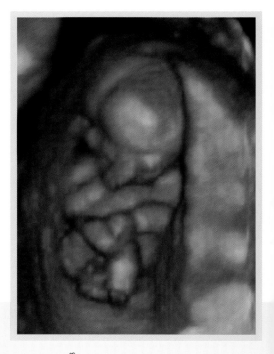

My face is looking more human; my eyes have moved closer together on my face and my ears are almost in their correct position. I can open and close my lips. My neck is strong enough to support head movements.

The first of my bone tissue has appeared and ribs can be distinguished. My liver is making bile, and my kidneys are secreting urine into my bladder.

Girl or Boy?

The embryonic sex organs in boys and girls remain identical in the early weeks although a baby's sex has already been genetically assigned. On scanning, the genital organs are indistinguishable until the third month of gestation. After week 8, external genitalia appear in both sexes in the form of a protrusion with a central groove. If the urethral groove remains open, then you are expecting a girl. If the groove closes up, you will have a boy. On scans, if the genitals stick up, it's a boy; if they point downward, it's a girl.

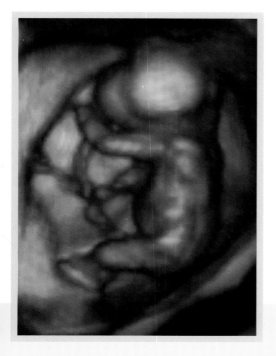

This little fetus is first viewed curled up at rest, then up and about playing with his umbilical cord.

The umbilical cord is baby's plaything and is often seen wrapped around a baby's neck or body. This is not a cause for alarm, as the cord is very elastic, and a baby cannot easily exert sufficient tension to block the cord's functions.

Week

GESTATION
12 weeks

LENGTH
3¼ to 4 inches (80 to 93 mm) from crown to rump

WEIGHT
1 ounce (25 g)

My movements are smoother now and I can bend, flex, and twist my fingers, hands, wrists, legs, knees, and toes. My nervous system has begun to function. Eyelids and fingernails and toenails continue to develop and I even have a sprinkling of hair on my head.

I'm starting to "practice" breathing movements although, as there is no air inside the uterus, all my oxygen

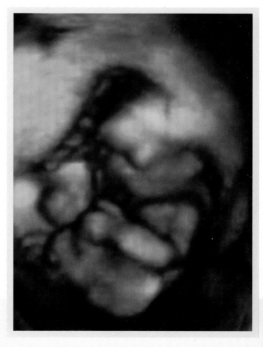

WEEK 14

comes via the umbilical cord from the placenta.

My neck is elongating so that my chin no longer rests on my chest. I have cheeks! My ears are further forward and are higher on my head. You can make out the bridge of my nose. My external genitalia are developing more definitely and it's getting easier to determine my sex.

The Fetal Heartbeat

At 6 weeks of pregnancy, fetal heart pulsations can be seen on ultrasound beating at 125 beats per minute (bpm). By 7 weeks, the rate is 150 bpm, and at 8 weeks, 175 bpm. By 16 weeks of pregnancy, the heart-rate has settled to between 120 and 160 bpm – about twice an adult's rate – which is the resting rate for the remainder of pregnancy. If you ask your midwife or doctor if you can listen to the heartbeat, you should be able to hear it from 16 weeks by means of a small Doppler probe. Many couples find this to be very reassuring. In labor, the heart-rate may be continuously monitored as an indication of fetal wellbeing.

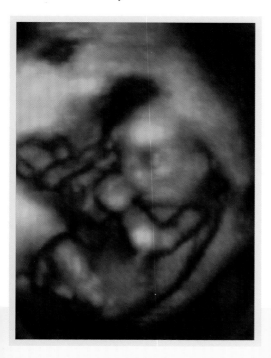

The thumb-sucking reflex develops early as this baby demonstrates. She is able to separate her thumb from her fingers – preparing for action – and then bring her thumb to her mouth.

Week

GESTATION
13 weeks

LENGTH
4 to 4½ inches (104 to 114 mm) from crown to rump

WEIGHT
1¼ ounce (50 g)

Although you can't see it, my skeleton is producing more bone. This helps my arms to bend at the wrist and elbow more easily. I can bend my fingers into fists although this is something that is not yet under the control of my brain.

A downy type of extra-fine hair, called *lanugo,* is starting to appear on my skin. This will help me to regulate my body temperature. This hair follows the pattern of my parchment-thin skin and creates patterns that look like

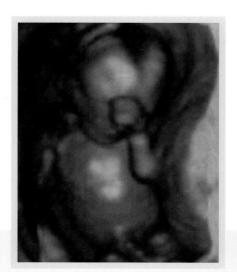
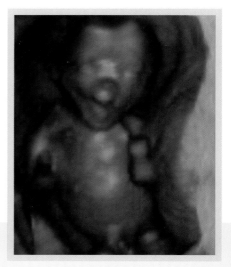

fingerprints over my body. I'm also acquiring eyebrows and there's more hair on my head.

The very small bones in my middle ear have begun to harden, but as my brain's auditory centers haven't developed yet, I don't know what it is I am hearing. I do, however, have a range of facial expressions: I can frown and grimace.

Limb development

The hands develop first and then the feet. Some scientists believe that this is because development follows use. As a baby will have to hold things prior to standing and walking, feet develop later. An alternative theory is that the hands develop earlier, along with the eyes and ears, because they, too, are sense organs.

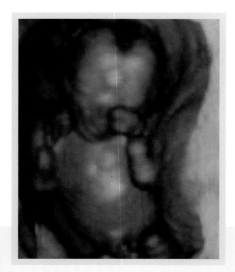

This little baby demonstrates a range of physical movements. He can move his hands, clench his fist, and yawn. He is perfecting those activities that will equip him for survival outside.

Week

GESTATION
14 weeks

LENGTH
4⅓ to 4⅔ inches (108 to
116 mm) from crown to
rump

WEIGHT
2¾ ounces (80 g)

My arms and legs are complete and
my legs are growing longer than my
arms. All my joints are working and
everything moves. What bones I
have are becoming harder and
retaining calcium.

Although I still have to rely on my
mother's antibodies, which cross the
placenta, my immune system can now
produce antibodies.

My nervous system is operating and
my muscles respond to stimulation
from my brain, so I can coordinate
my movements.

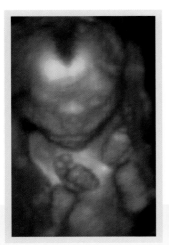 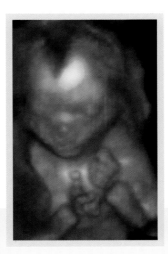 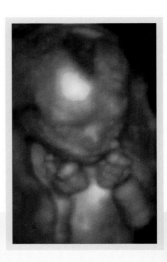

WEEK 16

This is quite an active time for me, and I enjoy rolling over, kicking, and somersaulting.

An ultrasound expert should be able to discern my sex easily. But what you may not see or feel is that I am occasionally hiccuping. These hiccups are noiseless because there is no air in my trachea, only fluid.

Amniocentesis

From this week, a fetus increases the number of cells he sheds into the amniotic fluid. These cells contain information about his chromosomes, and can be used to test for genetic abnormalities. The amniotic fluid cells are removed, incubated, and cultured; results can take 1-2 weeks. A more rapid test, Fluorescent in Situ Hybridization (FISH), takes only 24-48 hours. Although it doesn't give a detailed chromosome analysis (karyotype), it can detect major changes of chromosome numbers (such as found in Down's syndrome) and may be used if the likelihood of a chromosomal abnormality is high.

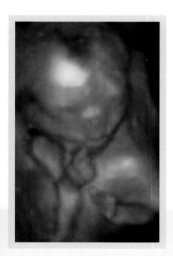
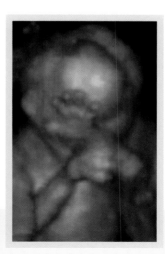

This baby demonstrates a great variety of movements within the space of a few seconds. He twists and turns his hands, clenches and extends his fingers, touches his face, and keeps his thumbs up in case the opportunity for sucking arises. The rapidity, subtlety, and complexity of these movements show an advanced degree of cerebellar control.

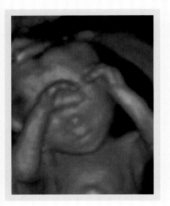 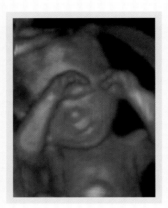 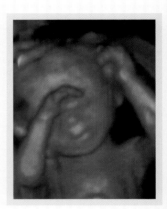

Defined as the unconscious sense of body-in-space, proprioception is dependent on a variety of information received by the brain from the ears, eyes, nose, and limbs. At around this stage of gestation, 17 weeks, the brain is developing the neural pathways that will enable a fetus to begin to sense the other parts of his body. Proprioception is a dynamic sense; it allows us to adopt to a shifting environment. The cerebellum is the fastest growing part of the brain at this time, and it governs this range of behavior.

Although proprioception won't fully mature until your baby is born and has his senses stimulated in a variety of ways, the first signs of it appear early in fetal development.

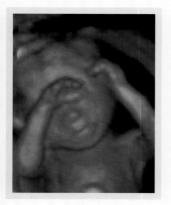 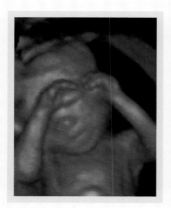 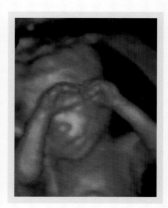

This baby begins to bring his hands together, but just as they get close, they spring apart – possibly a reflex action. He perseveres, however, and at last manages to bring his fingers together. Has he recognized another part of himself?

"Of all the clever people round me here, I most delight in Me"

Week

GESTATION
15 weeks

LENGTH
4½ to 5 inches (11 to 12 cm)
from crown to rump

WEIGHT
3½ ounces (100 g)

My head is beginning to look in proportion to the rest of my body but my face is thin due to its lack of subcutaneous fat. My eyes are still closed but they are much larger. I've got more hair on my head, eyebrows, and eyelashes, which have grown longer. I also have finger- and toenails.

I can do a lot with my hands, including putting them in my mouth. My fingers are very well developed; you can see all the individual phalanges (finger bones) in the pictures below.

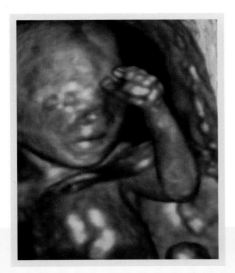
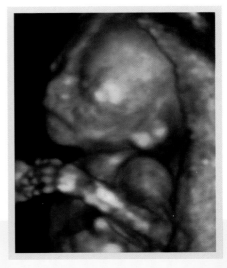

My circulatory and urinary systems are working perfectly. I remove amniotic fluid by swallowing and "top it up" from my bladder. My chest rises and falls as I practice breathing movements and amniotic fluid is passing into and out of my air passages (and out of my body as well). My heart pumps as much as 50 pints (24 liters) of blood a day. I'm beginning to acquire brown fat, which will help me to regulate my body heat once I'm born.

Amniotic fluid

Made up of fluid from the placenta and baby's lung and fetal urine, amniotic fluid peaks at about 2-2½ pints (1000-1200ml) at 36-38 weeks of pregnancy and then, inexplicably, falls off rapidly to about 10 ounces (300ml) at week 42. Babies begin to swallow amniotic fluid at around 19 weeks of gestation. Scientists believe they do so to aid the growth and development of the fetal digestive system and to help condition it to function after birth. Amniotic fluid also may contribute by providing essential nutrients. A full-term baby may swallow as much as 1¼ pints (500 ml) of it in a 24-hour period.

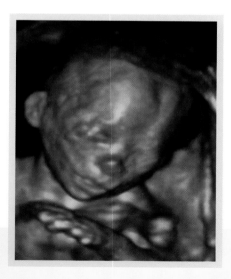

Though thin of face, this baby has beautifully formed ears, lips, nose, and chin. In a series of scans taken in rapid succession she is seen in constant movement, rotating her body and opening and closing her hands. You can see her individual phalanges (finger bones).

These scans also reveal much of the interior of the uterus. In the first picture, you can see the blood vessels of the uterine wall. In the second photo, the placenta is clearly visible behind the fetal head, while at the top of the third picture, you can see the lining of the womb.

Week

LENGTH
5 to 5½ inches (12.5 to 14 cm) from crown to rump

WEIGHT
5¼ ounces (150 g)

Possibly because she's acquired a bit more facial fat, this baby has a "cuter" look than last week's. There's a good view of the coronal and parietal sutures, the structures that keep the skull open while the brain is forming. She also exhibits a very unusual feature. Though most doctors believe the eyelids remain fused until week 24, this baby has at least one eye wide open!

Inside my fast-growing lungs, tiny air sacs called alveoli are beginning to develop. At this stage, however, they are only potential spaces and my respiratory system is among the last to mature.

Pads have formed on my fingertips and toes, and the unique swirls and whorls that will be my fingerprints begin to appear. I can maneuver my hands well, even getting them to my mouth. I also enjoy punching, kicking, turning, and wriggling.

My eyes are now in their correct position although the lids are thought to remain closed until week 24 in order to protect them.

Undigested debris from swallowed amniotic fluid is accumulating in my lower bowel. This paste-like material is called *meconium*. It will induce my first bowel movement.

As with other boy babies, my prostate is forming.

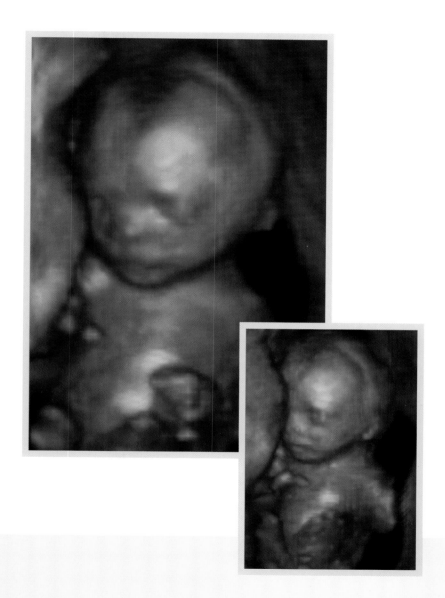

Week

GESTATION
17 weeks

LENGTH
5¼ to 6 inches (13 to 15 cm)
from crown to rump

WEIGHT
7 ounces (200 g)

*This fetus has his thumb poised
for sucking, though my series of
scans did not reveal whether or not
he actually got it into his mouth.
He also exhibits another frequently
seen phenomenon, that of having
the soles of his feet touch.*

Vernix caseosa, a thick, white greasy substance, is being secreted by glands in my skin and will act as a waterproof barrier to protect me.

Another fatty coating, *myelin*, is produced to coat my nerves. This insulates them and allows for the smooth, rapid exchange of information that will allow me to perform coordinated, skilful movements. Overall, however, I have a comparative lack of this substance, which is not fully present until I've matured from a newborn.

My gut is beginning to produce gastric juices that help me to absorb amniotic fluid and pass it into my circulation. My blood is then filtered by my kidneys and the fluid excreted back into the amniotic sac.

Nipples are starting to appear. If I'm a girl, my vagina, uterus, and fallopian tubes are in place. If I'm a boy, my genitals are distinct and recognizable.

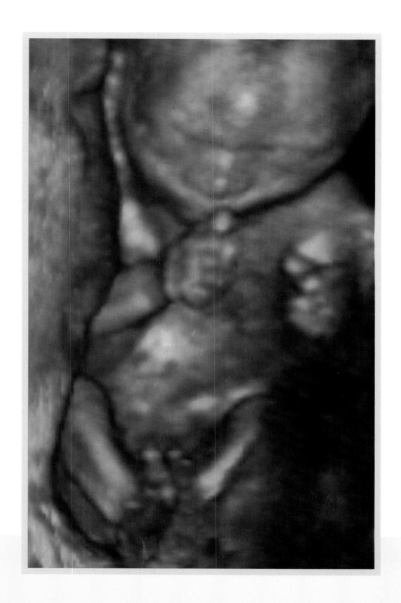

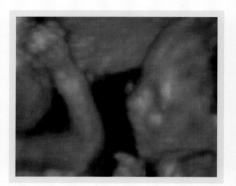
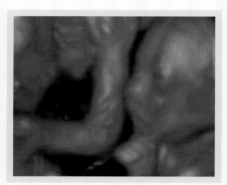

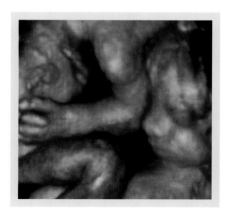

The uterine environment is a tricky one for twins. It encourages both companionship and competition for space.

Positively speaking, twins are often immensely sensitive to each other's needs, emotionally close and mutually consoling. But familiarity can breed contempt! In the sequence shown here, taken at 20 weeks, one twin looks as though he is giving his brother a clout but, thankfully, it all ends well.

Research done on twins in utero found that early contact between babies began at about 12 weeks of pregnancy and consisted of an action-reaction sequence. More complex behavior began, on average, at about 14 weeks, and consisted

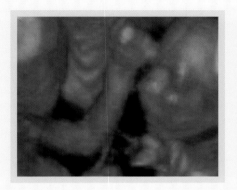
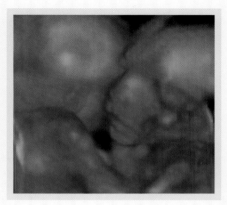

of close long-lasting contacts involving the legs, arms, mouths, and whole bodies. Interestingly, such "complex contacts" occurred earlier between female twins. Complex activities seem to correlate with the development of the brain's neural system. The study also suggested that activity itself promoted brain growth. Twins experience more tactile stimuli and they often perform better on certain developmental tests once born.

"So we two grew together, like to a double cherry, seeming parted, but yet an union in partition…"

Week

GESTATION
18 weeks

LENGTH
5½ to 6½ inches (14 to 16 cm) from crown to rump

WEIGHT
9 ounces (255 g)

I've reached the halfway mark in my development! Now is a crucial time for the development of my senses – taste, smell, hearing, sight, and touch. The nerve cells serving each of these are developing in their particular areas of my brain. There also is an increase in the complex connections required for the development of memory and thinking functions.

My skin is getting thicker; there are now four layers. One of these contains epidermal ridges, which are responsible for surface patterns on the fingertips, palms and soles of the feet. More vernix is accumulating. My heartbeat can be heard with a stethoscope.

If I'm a girl I already have about six million eggs in my ovaries. However, by the time I'm born, there will only be about a million.

The face of this fetus continues to mature. His nose is lengthening and his head seems more in proportion to his body.

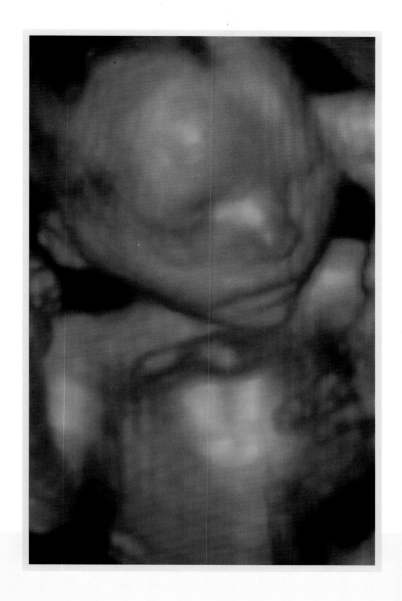

Week

LENGTH
7¼ inches (16 cm) from
crown to rump

WEIGHT
10½ ounces (about 300 g)

The extra weight I've been putting on will help me to keep warm after I'm born. I'm swallowing lots of amniotic fluid; this is good practice for my digestive system, which absorbs the water. Although my kidneys can remove some of the waste products, the rest are conveyed by the placenta to my mother's bloodstream and then to her kidneys.

Taste buds have formed on my tongue and my sense of touch keeps

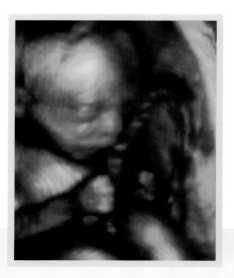
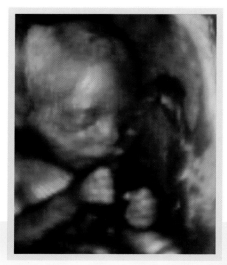

improving due to the development of my brain and nerve endings.

I often can be seen on ultrasound stroking my face, sucking my thumb, or playing with my umbilical cord.

Head Size

Your baby's head remains larger in proportion to the rest of his body until late in pregnancy. In week 13, your baby's head is about half of his crown-to-rump measurement. By week 21, your baby's head is about one-third of his overall body length. At birth, it will be about one-quarter the size of his body. When fetal head growth slows down, body growth accelerates.

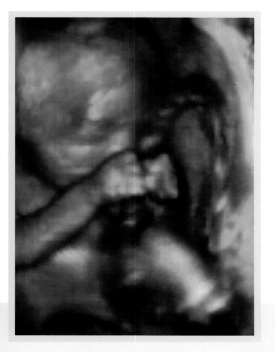

This baby is quite content to be clasping her umbilical cord. You see a clear view of it emerging from the placenta and arching downward. The umbilical cord generally sits in front of the baby. This baby brings her hands together in order to take hold of it.

WEEK 21

Week

GESTATION
20 weeks

LENGTH
7½ inches (19 cm) from
crown to rump

WEIGHT
12¼ ounce (350 g)

My brain has begun to grow very quickly now, especially the germinal matrix, a structure in the center of my brain that produces brain cells.

My skin is redder and less transparent but wrinkled and covered in lanugo. I have developed sweat glands. My fingernails are fully formed and continue to grow.

If I'm a boy, my testes have begun descending from my pelvis to my scrotum and primitive sperms have already formed. If I'm a girl, my vagina begins to hollow.

I'm awake more often and when I am, I can hear conversations, loud noises and music. I may even wake up if my mother taps on her abdomen.

This baby has achieved a unique look all his own. You can clearly see how well developed his ear is and there is a good view of his collarbone or clavicle.

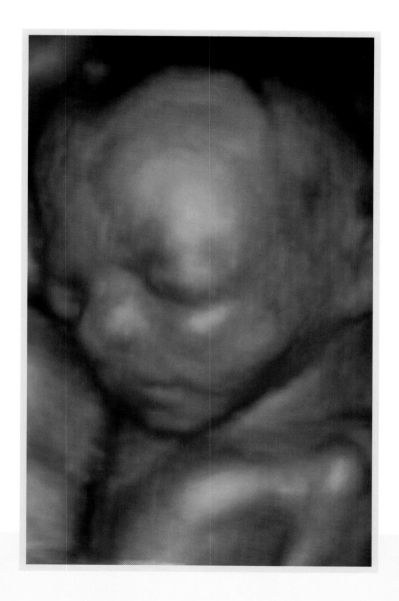

Week

GESTATION
21 weeks

LENGTH
8 inches (20 cm) from crown to rump

WEIGHT
1 pound (455 g)

Both my face and body are looking more and more like those of a full-term baby but my bones and organs are still a little visible beneath my skin. The latter, however, is becoming less transparent. Because I don't have much subcutaneous fat, my skin is still quite wrinkly. I have quite distinct lips and there are tooth buds beneath my gum line. My lanugo hair may be darker.

My hearing is much more acute now because the bones of my inner ear have hardened. Interestingly, I can hear my dad's deeper voice easier than I can hear my mother's higher pitched one.

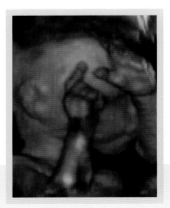
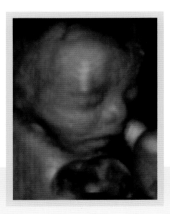
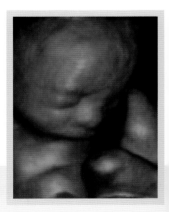

My eyes are formed but my iris (the colored part) still lacks pigment.

Internally, my pancreas is developing steadily; this will supply insulin, an important hormone for laying down fat in my tissues.

Hearing

The uterus is not a quiet place. A baby is privy to a wide range of sounds such as those made by her mother's voice, organs, and circulation; her burps, hiccups, and sneezes, as well as outside noises. From the 26th week of pregnancy onward, babies listen all the time when they are awake. They react to sounds by demonstrating the startle reflex – they fling their arms and legs out to their sides. While in the uterus, your baby already recognizes your voice – its individual qualities, tones, and rhythms, thus she also has the ability to distinguish language from other sounds.

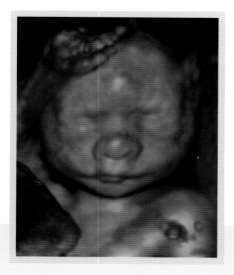

This baby demonstrates the very active nature of life in the second trimester. Her fingers can bend and straighten, she can bring her knees up, and she can stroke her head with her fingers.

WEEK 23

Week 24

GESTATION
22 weeks

LENGTH
8½ inches (21 cm) from crown to rump

WEIGHT
1¼ pounds (540 g)

This is a landmark week because, with expert care, it is now possible I can survive outside the uterus. I'm still very thin, however, and while I practice breathing by inhaling amniotic fluid, my lungs are still very immature. Airway passages form tubes in my lungs and blood vessels, and air sacs are starting to develop there. Of course, there is no air in the uterus so the air sacs are flattened. Even the fluid does not distend them. I'm also beginning to produce surfactant, the substance that keeps the air sacs from sticking together; this will help my lungs expand when I'm born.

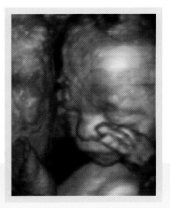
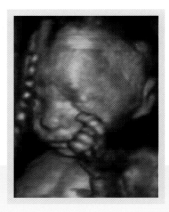
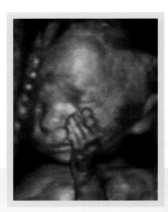

My face is filling out, and my eyelashes and eyebrows are well formed. While my head is still larger in proportion to my torso, the rest of my body is continuing to grow. I am beginning to build up fat but my skin remains red and wrinkled. The skin on my hands and feet is thicker than it is on the rest of my body.

At this time, my hearing is very well established. I can hear my mother's voice, her heartbeat, and her stomach rumblings! I particularly like it when she plays classical music.

Vernix

This is a thick, white, fatty substance, produced by the sebaceous glands, which develops during the last trimester of pregnancy. It helps to prevent a baby's skin from becoming waterlogged. Babies born prematurely have a lot of vernix on their skins, while overdue babies have virtually none at all. In some hospitals, the vernix is washed off after birth, while in others it is left to wear off naturally, usually within a few days. It is felt this offers a baby a measure of protection for a few days more.

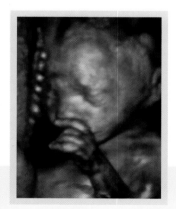 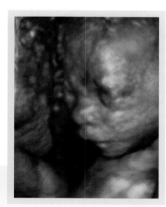

This handsome fellow can't seem to let himself alone! He rubs his eye, scratches and then pats his cheek, and rubs his nose. He seems a bit tired out at the end. Note the umbilical cord draped over his right eye.

WEEK 24

Trimester 3

In the third trimester (weeks 25-40), the baby puts on weight and perfects those behavioral patterns – sucking, swallowing, yawning, and grasping, which will prepare her for life outside the womb. During this time, your baby's weight will triple, and her length doubles. Whereas growth in the first two trimesters involved mainly cell division or hyperplasia, growth is now almost entirely by cell fattening or hypertrophy. Your baby is taking on stores of fat to help her keep warm, protein to build muscles and other tissues, calcium to develop her bones, and key nutrients such as iron to make her function correctly.

25 WEEKS PREGNANCY

Next to dramatic weight gain, there is also dramatic brain development. New cells and connections between cells form constantly. Much of brain growth is due to the laying down of myelin, a substance that coats the nerves and allows signals to move much more rapidly.

27 WEEKS PREGNANCY

A baby is considered full term when she has reached 38 weeks gestation, though from 36 weeks onward, most babies do well, with little specialist care. Babies born earlier than 34 weeks usually require medical intervention to survive, though more and more do so. Lung formation is generally not complete until late in the third trimester. The alveoli (future air sacs) do not expand until after birth but the surface tension in the alveoli gradually reduces as pregnancy progresses under the influence of surfactants, so that expansion of the lungs occurs as soon as the baby is born.

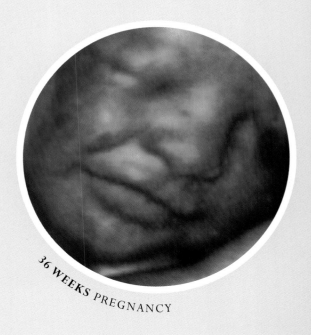

36 WEEKS PREGNANCY

Week 25

GESTATION
23 weeks

LENGTH
8¾ inches (22 cm) from
crown to rump

WEIGHT
1½ pounds (700 g)

I'm now more well proportioned
though still thin-skinned and skinny.
Blood vessels continue to develop in my
lungs and my nostrils begin to open.

High inside my gums, my
permanent teeth are developing in
buds. These won't descend until my
baby teeth start to fall out when I'm
six. The nerves around my mouth and
lip are more sensitive now – I think this

This fetus demonstrates true baby-like
features; the proportions of her face are
those of a mature baby. She's using her
umbilical cord as a pillow.

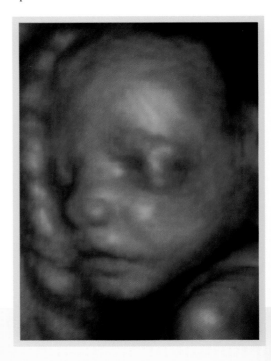

is to prepare me for the essential task of finding my mother's nipple once I'm born, so I can nurse.

Most of my vital organs are well developed except for my lungs. If I'm a girl, my vagina has become a hollow tube.

My umbilical cord is now thick and resilient and is my crucial lifeline.

The Umbilical Cord

This is a firm, protective, jelly-like cord, which contains two arteries and a vein that are coiled around each other. Blood rushes through it at a quick pace, keeping it distended so it doesn't get knotted or kinked. This means it is very unlikely to get obstructed even if it becomes wrapped around the baby's neck and because it is very strong, it can sustain squeezing and twisting by the baby. It is, in essence, your baby's lifeline, as it delivers oxygen and nutrients which have crossed the placenta from the mother's circulation through to the baby. Babies frequently grip their cords (see week 21), which, since they share the same environment, may be a source of consolation. The cord grows to about 22 inches (60 cm) in length in pace with your baby, enabling him or her to move freely in the uterus.

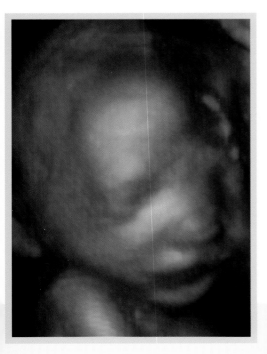

WEEK 25

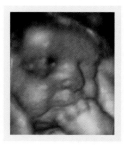

It's no wonder babies practice thumb-sucking in the uterus because sucking is among the most important survival skills they will have when they are born. Sucking one's thumb not only prepares a baby for being able to feed immediately after birth but helps her to use touch to explore the world.

While she's developing, your baby's mouth with its enormous number of nerve endings is a much more sensitive organ than her hands. Therefore, when she sucks her fingers, she also is learning about the feel of her skin, and the size and shape of her finger.

Thumb-sucking is practiced early in utero; fetuses as young as 11 weeks have been seen with their thumbs in their mouths. Older babies (see week 37), will suck any part of the body that comes near.

Most commonly the fetus will suck her thumb, as the 26-week-old fetus on the opposite page demonstrates. First she senses the top of her thumb with her lips, then the thumb is in her mouth for a proper suck. The 34-week-old fetus on the right has been captured starting out sucking his smaller toes and, finding them not quite to his liking, has gone on to suck a bigger and better toe.

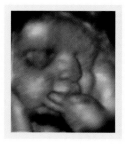

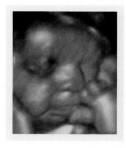

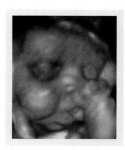

"O for a life of sensations rather than of thoughts!"

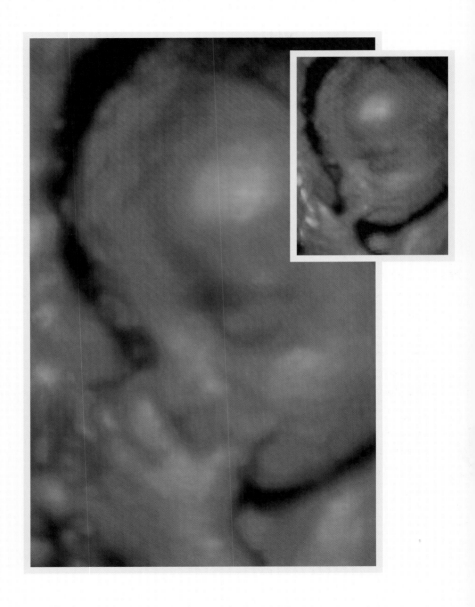

Week 26

GESTATION
24 weeks

LENGTH
9⅛ inches (23 cm) from crown to rump

WEIGHT
2 pounds (910 g)

My lungs are still maturing and while I still have some growing to do, the space in the uterus is becoming constricted.

My spine is getting stronger and more supple to support my growing body. I can hold my feet and curl my hand into a fist. My fingernails are all present and I have eyebrows and eyelashes. I make breathing movements even though there is no air in my lungs. This motion helps to mature my lungs so that they can expand at birth.

If I'm a boy, the cells in my testes, which make testosterone, have increased in number.

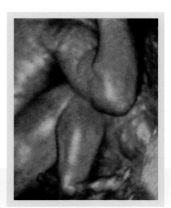 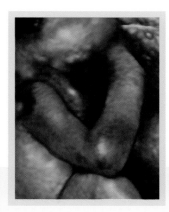 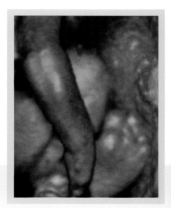

Although only specialist testing can reveal the reaction in my brain, I do respond to touch and sound. My pulse quickens when I hear something and I may even move in rhythm to music. If my dad puts his head to my mother's abdomen, he may be able to hear my heartbeat.

Reaction

Throughout this book and others, there are references to fetuses reacting and parents may want to know what is meant. Scientists use the following criteria as responses: A quickening or slowing down of the heartbeat; patterns of movements including kicks and the throwing out of arms and legs and rapid eye movement (REM).

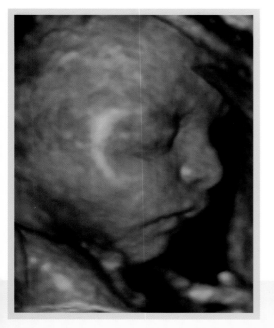

A scan at 26 weeks is truly a bonding experience. Parents are anxious to see as much of their baby's anatomy as they can before birth while it is still possible. Here, we have a good view of this baby's elbow and knee, hand under his foot, and mobile fingers. He also demonstrates a beautiful profile.

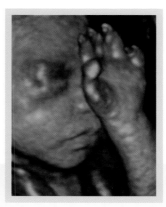

WEEK 26

Week

GESTATION
25 weeks

LENGTH
9½ inches (24 cm) from crown to rump and 15 inches (38 cm) long with legs extended

WEIGHT
2 pounds 2 ounces (1 kg)

Eye Color

Most Caucasian babies are born with dark blue eyes. Eye pigmentation needs light exposure to complete its formation, and the true eye color may not be apparent for weeks or months. Dark-skinned babies usually have dark gray or brown eyes at birth, developing into a true brown or black after the first six months or a year.

The long development of my eyes is now complete as the final layers of my retina in the back of my eye have now formed. My eyelids, which previously were fused, can now open some of the time. My eyelashes, too, are fully grown. They help to protect my delicate eyeballs from harmful matter now and will continue to do so once I'm born.

I'm becoming more rounded and plumper due to increased amounts of fat being deposited under my skin. My lungs continue to grow and I have fully functioning taste buds on my tongue and inside my cheeks.

This baby has a mature face with recognizable features. The cord is just visible pressing up against his chest.

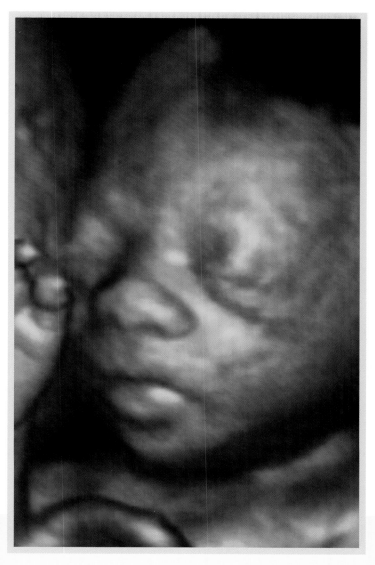

WEEK 27

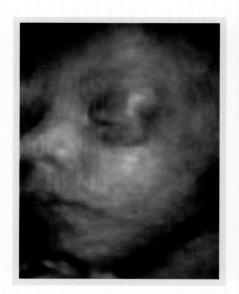
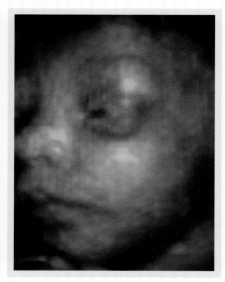

"Was it a vision, or a waking dream?... Do I wake or sleep?"

Although many books on fetal development claim that unborn babies can blink, what sonographers actually see is a baby opening and closing his eyelids.

While your baby's eyes are developing, his eyelids remain closed to allow his retinas to develop. At about 24 weeks, retinal development is complete and his eyelids begin to open.

Although it is dark in the uterus, a baby will go through intermittent periods when his eyes will open, though most of the time they will be closed. By 33 weeks, his pupils will be capable of constricting and dilating so that he can make out dim shapes.

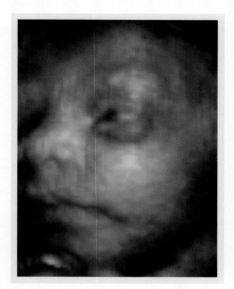 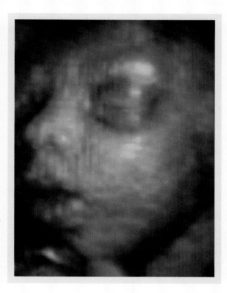

Practice opening and closing the eyelids will help him perfect the blinking reflex. Once he's born, this will protect his eyes against approaching objects, shield his delicate corneas from harmful light, and keep his eyes moist. A newborn will automatically close his eyes if something makes contact with the bridge of his nose, or if he is startled by a bright light or loud noise, or even if he just feels a rush of air on his face.

Many reflexes that your baby is born with will disappear over time but the blinking reflex remains with us for life. Perhaps it also is practice for the visual stimulation that is all around us once we're born.

This fetus of 27 weeks is seen opening and closing his eyelids over a period of two seconds.

Week 28

GESTATION
26 weeks

LENGTH
10 inches (25 cm) from
crown to rump

WEIGHT
2½ pounds (1.1 kg)

I'm about one-third of my estimated birth weight and although I would find it very difficult to breathe properly unaided if I was born now, my lungs are capable of breathing air. I do have periods when I make regular breathing movements but the fluid only enters the main air passages (bronchi) and not my lungs. The movement of fluid may help the development of the alveoli (future

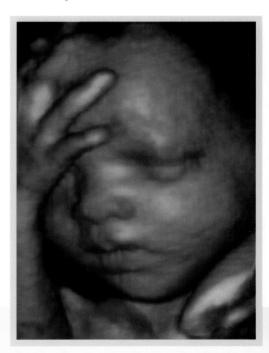

Speak to me
Babies at this time enjoy hearing their parents' voices, so remember to talk to your baby from time to time. Singing a lullaby is another way to keep in touch with your baby.

air sacs). Sometimes I have hiccups, which my mother may feel as small intermittent jerks.

My skin is red and now completely covered by vernix, a protective greasy coating. Baby fat is accumulating underneath my skin and my muscles are becoming well developed. I also am now developing scalp hair, especially on the back of my head. The network of nerves to my ear is now complete and I'm hearing more and enjoying the experience. I also like to suck my thumb or my fingers.

If I'm a boy, my testes have nearly finished their descent into my scrotum. If I'm a girl, my labia are still small and don't yet cover my clitoris. The labia will grow closer together in the last few weeks of pregnancy.

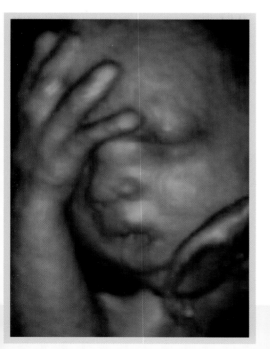

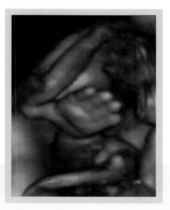

The accumulation of fat has resulted in this fetus having chubby cheeks and well-formed lips. Fat also makes the skin creases on her fingers and palm much more evident. It is common for fetuses to keep their hands to their foreheads for extended periods of time.

WEEK 28

Week 29

GESTATION
27 weeks

LENGTH
10½ inches (26 cm) from crown to rump; almost 17 inches (43 cm) with legs extended

WEIGHT
2 pounds 12 ounces (1.25 kg)

It's becoming harder to find room to move around as I have done before though I still manage to stretch, flex and extend my legs and arms, and occasionally, get in a few kicks. Normally my mother will feel more than ten distinct kicks in the course of a morning. As I put on weight, my head becomes more in proportion to the rest of my body.

The big news is how much my brain is developing. It is growing quickly and the soft bones of my skull easily can expand to accommodate it. The surface of my brain is becoming more and more irregular as grooves and indentations

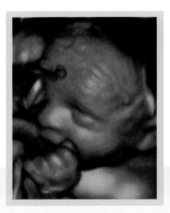
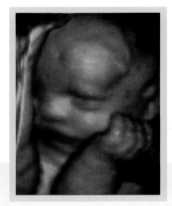
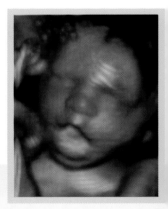

form. These are known as *gyri* and *sulci* and are a result of connections being built up between nerve cells. My brain is pretty powerful; it can control my breathing and body temperature, although I would still need the help of an incubator if born at this stage.

My senses also seem much more responsive. The lenses of my eyes move during periods of quiet sleep. They also are more sensitive to light although, as my surroundings are dark, this ability won't be put into play until I am born. Sounds, tastes, and smells also are more noticeable. The hair on my head is growing longer.

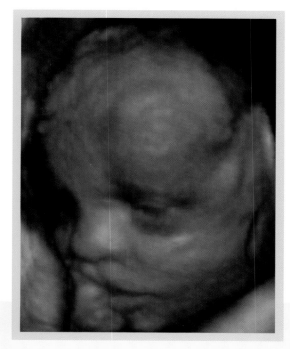

Although space is becoming restricted, this fetus still can move vigorously. In the third picture she is seen sticking her tongue out. Her skull bones are expanding to accommodate her growing brain while her eyes have opened momentarily. Most babies' eyes stay open from a fraction of a second up to about two seconds.

WEEK 29

Week 30

GESTATION
28 weeks

LENGTH
10¾ inches (27 cm) from crown to rump; 17 inches (43 cm) from head to toe

WEIGHT
3 pounds (1.36 kg)

The hair (lanugo) that covered my body is disappearing. A few fuzzy patches may be left at birth but they will rub off over the following weeks. The hair on my head is thicker.

My skin looks less wrinkled because I've laid down more baby fat. I'm looking a lot rounder and my fingernails and toenails are growing.

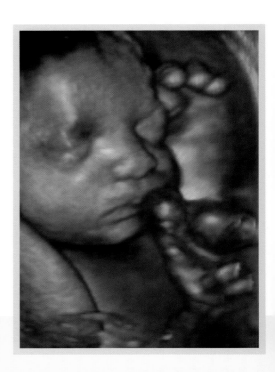

This baby's face is now developing a chubby newborn appearance due to increasing fat deposition. The umbilical cord normally floats in front of the face and is becoming thicker and stiffer.

My bone marrow has completely taken over the task of red blood cell production from my liver. My skeleton is hardening more and more, and my brain, muscles, and lungs continue to mature.

If I'm a girl, my clitoris is relatively prominent because my labia are still small and haven't covered it yet.

If I hear a noise, I will react to it with a kick. I increasingly open and close my eyes and I can breathe rhythmically.

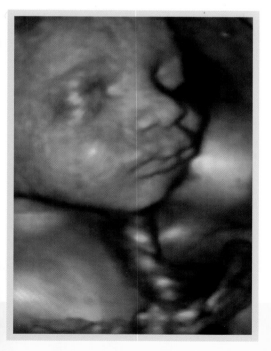

Memories

Between her 28th and 32nd week of gestation, the neural circuits in your baby's brain are as advanced as in a newborn's. At the same time, her cerebral cortex matures enough to support consciousness. This means that your baby is capable of feeling and remembering.

One recent study carried out to test memory exposed infants in utero to the theme tune of a soap opera. When they heard the same tune two to four days after birth, these babies reacted to the music (see page 71 for a description of reaction). The control group, which hadn't been played the tune in utero, made no response.

WEEK 30

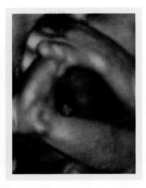

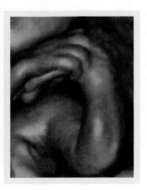

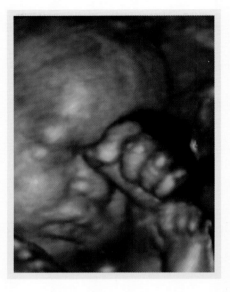

Grasping is one of the vital reflexes with which babies are born. It begins quite early but becomes better established during the third trimester. A newborn's grasp can be so strong that you could almost lift him up by his arms. And, if you try and remove your finger, his grip may tighten.

There are several well recognized patterns. One of the most common forms is the grasping of hands (see picture bottom left). Generally, newborn babies, and by association, unborn babies, grasp with their pinky fingers as the sequence above demonstrates. It is only later that an opposable thumb is employed. However,

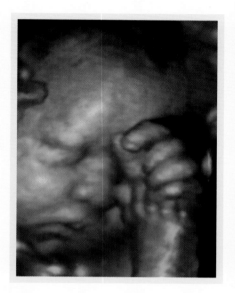 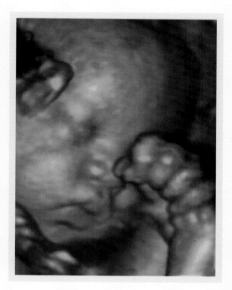

the baby shown above left is definitely precocious as he
can be seen grasping his foot with his thumb. In
addition to hands, feet, fingers, and toes, babies most
commonly grab hold of their umbilical cords and, in
the case of twins, they grab hold of each other.

"In gentleness of heart, with
gentle hand, Touch"

Week

GESTATION
29 weeks

LENGTH
11¼ inches (28 cm) from
crown to rump

WEIGHT
3½ pounds (1.59 kg)

I continue to put on weight but most of me is fully mature except for my lungs and digestive tract. My brain is constantly adding connections. My eyes are showing some color now, but their real color won't show until I'm six to nine months old. However, my eyes are being prepared for life after birth. My eyelids are frequently open during active times and closed during sleep.

Babies differ in their expressiveness; some, like this baby, have very mobile faces and others rarely change expression. This baby also keeps his hands quite busy, running them constantly over his face.

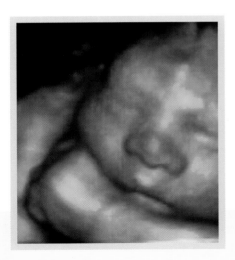 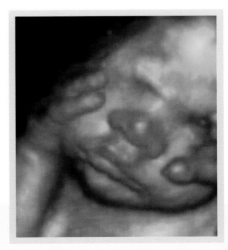

Behavior Patterns

Unborn babies are asleep for most of the time. However sleep alternates between quiet sleep, when few movements occur, and active (REM) sleep when the eyes move, body movements occur intermittently, and the heart-rate speeds up in response to this movement. In the last few weeks of pregnancy, the fetus alternates these sleep states in a cyclical fashion, about 30 per cent of the time being spent in quiet sleep and 60 per cent in active sleep. For about 10 per cent of the time the fetus is "awake" when there will be continuous movements of the body and limbs, the eyes will be moving, and the heart-rate will be fast. It is during this time that the face of the baby will be very expressive and yawning, blinking, and sucking will occur. All of these activities are preparing the baby for survival after birth. The fetus starts to make breathing movements as early as the first trimester. These movements help in the development of the lungs and prepare the chest muscles to take the first breath after the birth of the baby. It is the only activity which the baby carries out when in quiet sleep.

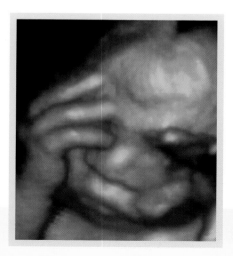 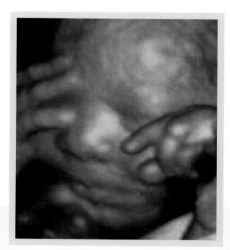

WEEK 31

Week 32

GESTATION
30 weeks

LENGTH
11½ inches (29 cm) from
crown to rump

WEIGHT
4 pounds (1.8 kg)

I can see, hear, taste, smell, and touch! My arms, legs, and body are continuing to fill out and they are proportional in size to my head.

My internal organs continue to mature. I'm breathing a lot, of course still only water, which helps my lungs to strengthen and develop. I'm also passing urine from my bladder.

My toenails are complete and I'm still growing hair on my head. If I'm a boy, my testes have finished their journey and both testicles are now in my scrotum.

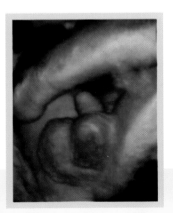
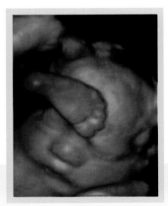
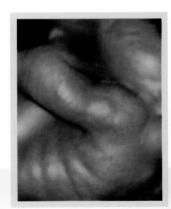

I sleep about 90 to 95 per cent of the day, but when I'm awake I move vigorously and open and close my eyes. Even when I'm sleeping, I perform certain activities (dream or REM sleep) when my eyeballs will move, and I will make breathing movements.

In preparation for birth I have now turned head-down in the uterus. I can still, however, kick upward under my mother's ribcage while my head is pressing on her pelvic floor. She may find this pretty uncomfortable!

Dreaming

At about 32 weeks gestation, rapid eye movement (REM), associated with dreaming, can be detected. Dreaming encourages a fetus's brain to develop; which is why a baby may spend the majority of his time sleeping. Perhaps a baby dreams of what he does during the day – moving his feet and hands, hearing sounds, and sharing emotional experiences with his mother.

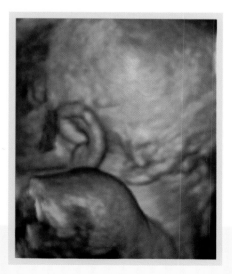

There's a lot to see on this baby including his genitals, his perfectly formed foot, his well-muscled body and the hair on the back of his head next to a beautifully formed ear.

WEEK 32

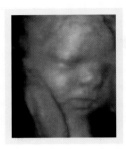

While in the uterus, babies spend most of their time sleeping. But this time isn't wasted. During periods of quiet and deep sleep, your baby is continually developing, growing, and preparing for birth. But some of the time a baby sleeps, her brain is working away and her eyes respond with little reflex movements, known as rapid eye movements or REM. This kind of sleep is associated with dreaming in adults but we can't be sure whether babies dream and if they do – of what.

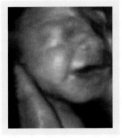

But we now can see that babies yawn. This 29-week-old fetus demonstrates that she has mastered the ability to produce a full, hearty yawn. In fact, she began yawning as early as 12 weeks of pregnancy. Is it in response to feelings of tiredness, could it be a sign of boredom, or is she simply perfecting her repertoire of gestures? In adults, yawns oxygenate blood by expanding and aerating the alveoli, or tiny lung sacs, and expelling carbon dioxide. Your baby, however, will only breathe once she's born, so maybe this behavior is nature's way of ensuring that as soon as your baby is delivered, she will be able to draw in all the air she needs to get her lungs and respiratory system working.

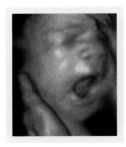

"A little sleep,
        a little slumber…"

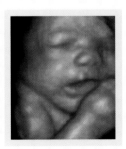

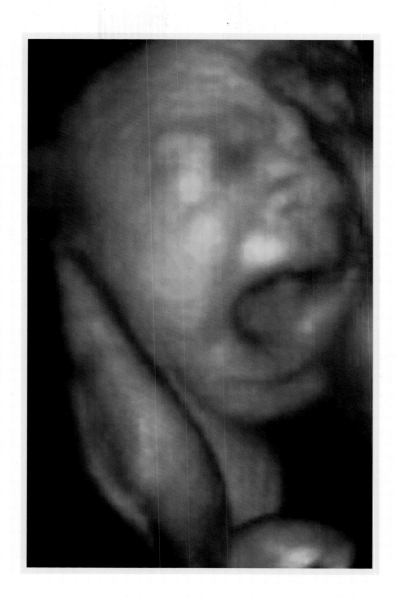

Week 33

GESTATION
31 weeks

LENGTH
12 inches (30 cm) from crown to rump, 19½ inches (43 cm) from head to toe

WEIGHT
4½ pounds (2 kg)

Due to rapid brain growth, my head circumference now has increased by about ⅜ inch (9.5mm) and is in the correct proportion to my body.

My bones are fully developed but still soft and pliable and I'm starting to store iron, calcium, and phosphorus, which are all important to further bone development.

The mechanism that controls my body temperature is beginning to function and while I am making rhythmic breathing movements, my lungs are not yet fully mature.

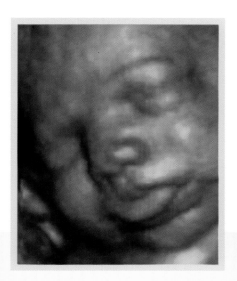
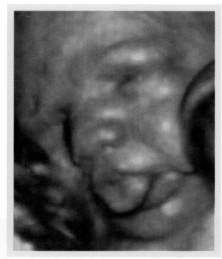

My skin is pinker and I'm accumulating much more fat.

I am increasingly aware of my surroundings, including external noises, and of my immediate environment such as the amniotic fluid.

Birth weight

In developed countries, babies average 7½ pounds (3.4 kg) at the end of a normal pregnancy lasting 40 weeks. About ⅓ of the eventual birth weight is reached by 28 weeks, ½ by 31 weeks, and ⅔ by 34 weeks. At one time it was thought a baby's growth slowed before term but now it is known that steady growth occurs up to and beyond 40 weeks. The baby's birth weight is almost entirely under the control of the mother; the father's genetic influence counts for very little. The heavier and taller the mother, the bigger will be the baby's birth weight. Boys are bigger than girls and second babies are bigger than first-borns. Asian babies are on average 6½ ounces (185g) and Afro-Caribbean babies are 4½ ounces (130g) lighter than Caucasian babies.

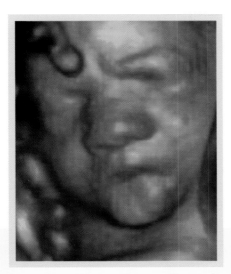

It is not unusual to see fetuses sticking out their tongues, and this behavior is more common in fetuses than newborns. This baby could be "tasting" the flavors of the amniotic fluid, which differ depending on what his mother has been eating and drinking.

WEEK 33

Week 34

Music

From now, your baby can recognize a particular piece of music and coordinate her movements in time with it. Classical music, particularly choral music and piano, have patterns closest to human speech, and are especially enjoyable for a baby. Depending upon the type of music heard, your baby may become stimulated and excited or sedated and relaxed.

My immune system is developing rapidly; it can help me fight mild infection. Although the tips of my fingers are very tiny, my fingernails have reached there and they are quite sharp.

My skin is less wrinkled and the color is becoming pinker. I still have quite a lot of vernix visible on my body.

While the rest of the bones in my body are hardening, my skull bones can still move quite freely over each other (called molding). This will enable me to ease out of the birth canal more easily.

It's difficult for me to float about in the amniotic fluid. I make fewer movements though they are more powerful and sustained. Unlike most babies at 34 weeks, I have not yet turned but hope to do so in the next two weeks.

You can see quite easily that this beautiful baby has a good amount of head hair. The umbilical cord partially covers his face, which is common with breech babies (see page 103).

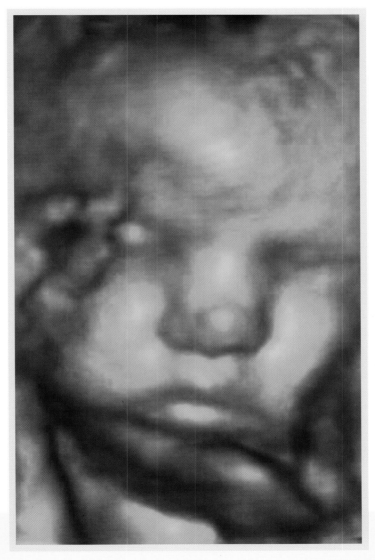

WEEK 34

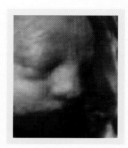

Although it has been claimed that crying has been heard inside the uterus, this has not been proved scientifically. When you cry you push air out of your lungs, but there is no air in the uterus and no air in a baby's lungs. But babies definitely show unhappiness and displeasure.

Sometimes, during a scanning procedure, when I've gently manipulated a baby to give her parents a better view on screen, the baby will make similar faces to this one. This baby is definitely grumpy and complaining about being awoken or moved out of position.

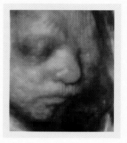

Doctors debate whether or when very young fetuses feel pain or discomfort and test for raised heartbeat and cortisol levels, which are classic signs. On the basis of these pain-detecting tests, it is now believed that fetuses feel pain at 24 weeks gestation. Now, with 4-D scanning, I think you can tell by just looking at their expressions.

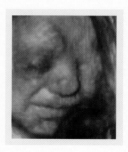

"But we…feel the heartbreak in the heart of things"

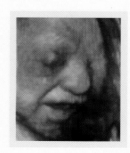

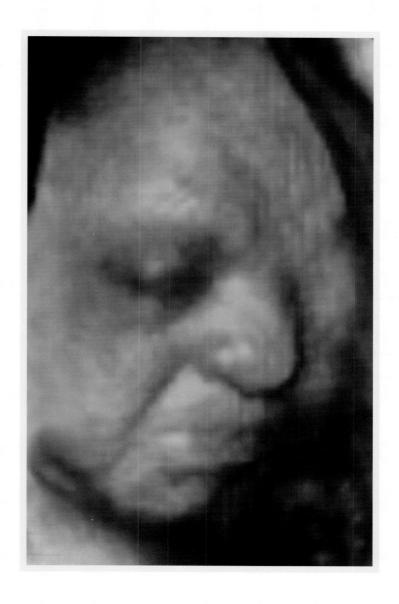

Week

GESTATION
33 weeks

LENGTH
13¼ inches (33 cm) from
crown to rump

WEIGHT
5½ pounds (2.55 kg)

*This baby's head has become engaged
in the birth canal – and you can see
what he thinks about his impending
entrance into the world!*

I'm getting plumper and plumper as I
acquire more body fat, which will later
help to regulate my body temperature.
There's hardly room to move around.

My central nervous system is
maturing, and I'm increasingly awake
and aware. My digestive system is
almost complete, and my lungs are
nearly fully mature.

Breathing

Your baby's lungs are the last major
organ to mature. In the latter weeks,
as your baby breathes, he or she
produces surfactant, a protein that's
essential for the lungs' healthy
development. Most babies' lungs are
not mature until at least 34 weeks of
pregnancy. A test which measures the
surfactant (LS-ratio) will provide an
index of fetal-lung maturation.
Maturation is signaled when the
amount of lecithin in the amniotic
fluid increases, and the amount of
sphingomyelin decreases.

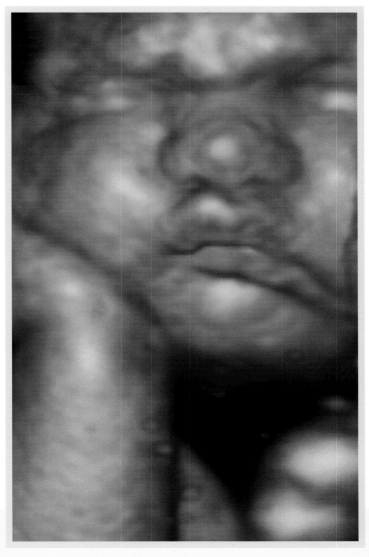

WEEK 35

If babies can show displeasure with a grimace (see page 94), doesn't smiling reveal inner contentment? This little baby is capable of cracking a wide grin.

Smiling is remarkable in that it's the only one of the behaviors developing babies exhibit that isn't demonstrated immediately after birth. Babies don't smile for at least 4-6 weeks post birth. It's understandable to think why a baby would smile in utero – she is warm and comfortable, she's never hungry, and she's shielded from loud noise and bright light, and reassured by the constant sound of her mother's heartbeat. Once a baby is born, she's thrust into a bright and noisy environment; she gets hungry; she feels cold and hot, and her nether region gets damp and soiled. No wonder, even as adults, we often long to return to the womb.

"Her loveliness I never knew, until she smiled at me…"

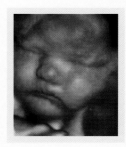

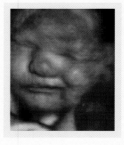

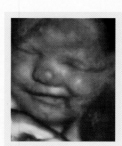

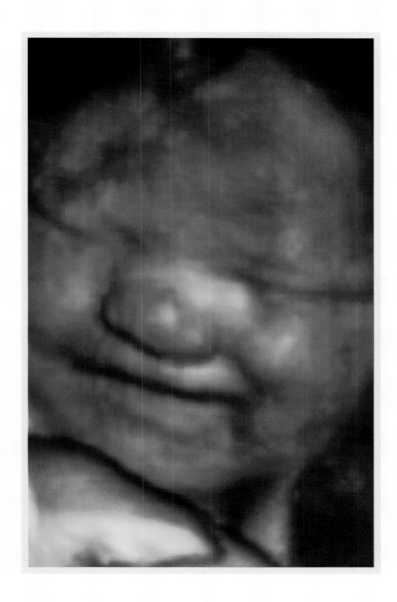

Week 36

GESTATION
34 weeks

LENGTH
13½ inches (34 cm) from
crown to rump; 18 to 20
inches (45 to 50 cm) with
legs extended

WEIGHT
6 pounds (2.75 kg)

I've pretty much reached my length at birth. Space is certainly getting tight and while I can still get in a good strong kick, I can't move around as much as I used to. Most of my time is spent putting on weight; I'll probably add half a pound this week.

I am awake for longer periods of time and this is reflected in a greater range of facial expressions.

My kidneys are now fully developed and my liver is able to process some

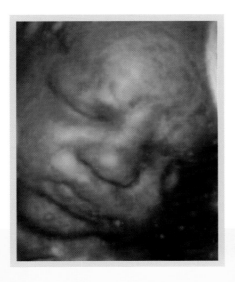
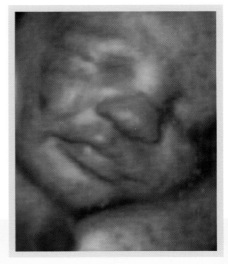

waste products. My fingernails now completely cover the tips of my fingers.

My face is smoothed out and if I have a raised birthmark, you might be able to see it now.

Bonding

Mother and child become attached to one another before birth. In providing nutrients and the chemicals that cause upset or pleasure, a mother creates a physiological bond. By rubbing her stomach in a reassuring way, she exhibits behavioral bonding. Some scientists also believe that mothers communicate sympathetically with their unborn babies, through dreams, for example.

Bonding is important following delivery because it determines a long-term emotional and affectionate relationship between mother and baby. Frequently, bonding does not immediately occur after birth and may take time to develop. 4-D ultrasound improves this process; it makes it easier for parents to establish a loving relationship prenatally that strengthens when the baby is born.

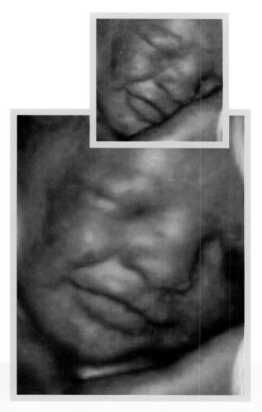

Initially, this fetus frowns but then apparently she has a happy thought resulting in a wide smile. Her skin is still covered with vernix but much of it is now floating in the amniotic fluid and can be seen on the picture on the left.

WEEK 36

Week

GESTATION
35 weeks

LENGTH
14 inches (35 cm) from crown to rump; 19 inches (47 cm) head to foot

WEIGHT
6½ pounds (2.95 kg)

From now on, I can be born almost at any time although no one knows what definitely triggers labor. Some scientists even suspect that secretions from my adrenal glands help to initiate the process.

I spend my time putting on weight and growing a bit in length.

My brain continues to develop. I can't kick like I used to but I can and do squirm a lot trying to stretch my arms and legs.

Most of the lanugo has disappeared but I have head hair, which varies from a few strands on the back of my head to a thick mop about an inch long.

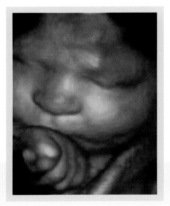

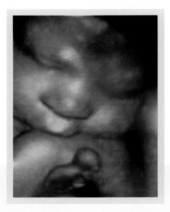

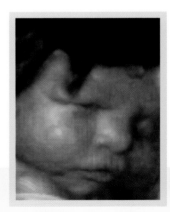

My immune system is still rapidly developing in order to protect me once I'm outside of the uterus. Those antibodies I do not produce myself, I receive from my mother via the placenta so, during the early weeks after birth, I am protected against infection.

Breech birth

The normal presentation for a baby is cephalic (head down) and this is associated with the least problems for delivery. Babies who do not turn head down present by the breech (bottom down). Breech deliveries are more complicated and most obstetricians nowadays will prefer to deliver a breech baby by Cesarean section, especially if it is a first baby. 40 percent of babies present by the breech at 26 weeks; 20 percent at 30 weeks; 10 percent at 34 weeks and 3 percent at term. Some obstetricians will try to help the baby turn (external version) at 36 weeks if the pregnancy is uncomplicated.

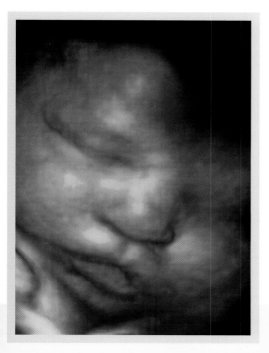

This baby seems both anxious to leave the womb and content to stay. In the first two pictures he is eagerly sucking his fist and the back of his arm. In the third picture he opens his eyes. But then he seems to drift off to sleep again. The dark area at the top of the pictures is the pelvic girdle. In actuality, he's already upside down waiting to be born.

WEEK 37

Weeks

GESTATION
38 weeks

LENGTH
14¾ to 15¼ inches (37 to 38 cm) crown to rump; total length 21½ inches (48 cm)

WEIGHT
7 pounds (3.25 kg)

I am clinically mature and can be born at any time. My abdominal circumference is now slightly larger than my head and I have about 15 per cent body fat. All my body systems have developed. My intestines have been accumulating meconium, which is a greenish-black sticky substance that is waste material. Some of this is lanugo, the soft hair that had previously covered my body.

I have more bones than my parents, who have 206, as some of mine will fuse together after I'm born and I grow.

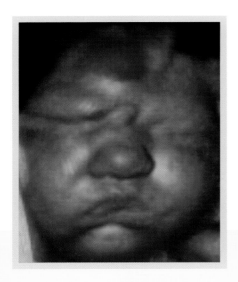

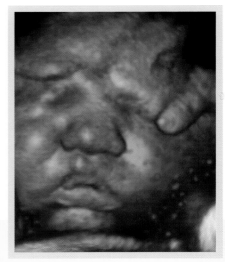

I have over 70 different reflexes to help me cope with the world outside the uterus.

The placenta, which has sustained me this many weeks, is now ageing, and becoming less efficient at transferring nutrients. There is less amniotic fluid, and the umbilical cord, which is about the same length as me, soon will finish its work. When I am born and take my first breaths of air, this process will trigger changes in the structure of my heart and arteries in order to divert blood to my lungs.

Being Born

Regular tightening and flexing of the uterus, or contractions, are a frequent occurrence in the latter part of the third trimester. These contractions are painless but help to cause thinning of the cervix and lower segment of the uterus so that the baby's head can descend into the pelvis.

Painful regular contractions, more frequent than one in ten minutes, are associated with labor, when the cervix actually dilates so that just before birth it is fully dilated, i.e. the uterus and vagina become one cavity. The muscles of the uterus now shorten to push the baby out with a little help from his or her mother.

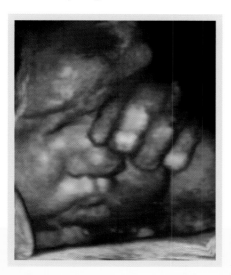

This baby doesn't seem very happy about the lack of space in his surroundings. Fortunately, he won't be inside much longer! The dark areas in the pictures are the shadows cast by the pelvic girdle. His head is fully engaged and he is actually facing downward.In the last weeks of pregnancy, babies' faces are increasingly expressive.

WEEK 38   WEEK 39   WEEK 40

What is an ultrasound scan exactly?
An ultrasound scan involves transmitting short pulses of high frequency but low intensity sound waves through the uterus. The frequency of the sound wave is above the limit of the human ear, so the baby will not hear the sound. The sound waves bounce off the baby and the returning echoes are translated by a computer into an image on a screen that reveals the baby's position and movements. Bone and other hard tissues are white in the image because they reflect the biggest echoes; organs and

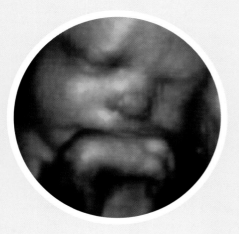

other soft tissues appear gray and speckled; while amniotic and other fluids appear black because they do not reflect any echoes at all. The sonographer looks at the contrast between these different shades of white, gray, and black to interpret the images.

Are there different types of ultrasound scans?
There are two ways of performing obstetrical ultrasounds – trans-abdominally and trans-vaginally. The first procedure is most useful in the second and third trimester. The ultrasound technician will put gel on your abdomen to facilitate the transmission of sound. Then he or she will move a transducer over your uterus to create pictures of your baby. Trans-vaginal ultrasound is used most commonly in the first trimester to give a very clear picture of the baby. Here, a transducer in the form of a long narrow probe, covered with a condom for sterility, will be placed in your vagina. The condom-coated transducer is

covered with gel for both lubrication and the transmission of sound waves. Neither form should be painful.

Does scanning harm my baby in any way?

Obstetric ultrasound was first used in 1958. Most developed countries have offered routine ultrasound as part of antenatal care for over 25 years. In some countries, two or three routine scans are offered. Literally, tens of millions of babies have been scanned and as yet, no risks have been demonstrated. Most regulatory bodies (like the FDA) while recognizing that ultrasound has never been shown to be harmful, recommend that ultrasound should only be used for medical purposes and that the sound output of the equipment should be within certain safety limits.

Who can perform an ultrasound?

Scans are usually performed by radiographers who are specially trained in ultrasound, and are known as sonographers. Most have completed a

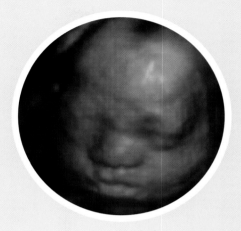

postgraduate training in medical ultrasound. If a special scan is required, say for a better view of the heart for a suspected problem, this will probably be done by a doctor known as a fetal medicine specialist.

What are the medical reasons for having an ultrasound scan?

If your due date is unclear; if there is vaginal bleeding or severe abdominal pain; if the uterus seems too big or too small when measured manually during prenatal visits; if there is a great risk of poor fetal growth or if growth can't be assessed adequately — say if a mother is

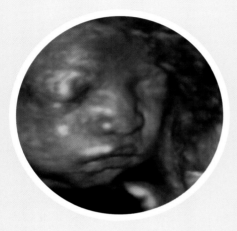

their baby as being more active, more beautiful, and more familiar. Additionally, after a scan, expectant mothers usually consider themselves more relaxed and less fearful.

With 3-D scans particularly, parents feel that they are meeting their baby for the first time. Fetal movement is very important; any demonstration of fetal behavior is more precious to the parents than even the most beautiful still photo.

overweight or is carrying twins; if there is an increased likelihood of birth defects, and in any situation where getting a clear image of the baby, placenta, uterus, or cervix will assist in the care of the mother and/or baby.

Besides checking that the baby is growing and developing normally, are there other benefits of having a scan?

Ultrasounds have been found to be a reassuring experience for parents and induce a positive attitude toward their growing baby. Even after just a single ultrasound, most parents perceived

Can my expected date of delivery change according to evidence on an ultrasound?

Early ultrasounds, those done in the first trimester, are extremely accurate at predicting gestational age. Only if your scan reveals that your baby measures more than three to four days from what your last menstrual period would suggest, would your due date change. Scans done in the second trimester are less accurate in establishing or confirming your due date, and those done in the third trimester are not accurate at all.

My caregiver examined my uterus and thinks that my pregnancy is more advanced. Might my baby come early?

If you have had an early scan, then it is the best predictor of the delivery date.

I'm told my baby is small. Is this not a good thing, because it will mean an easy birth?

Most small babies are perfectly healthy and yes, the birth is often easier. However, sometimes slow growth is due to poor circulation in the placenta and reduced transfer of oxygen and nutrients from a mother to her baby. Your obstetrician should be able to determine if your baby is small and healthy or growth-restricted, following a detailed ultrasound and Doppler examination. If your baby is growth-restricted, there is a high chance of an early delivery and cesarean section but the outcome is usually very good.

I've heard the phrase "ultrasound markers." What are these?

These are slight deviations from the normal anatomy seen on scan, which may or may not indicate a problem. While most are of no significance, some may indicate a chromosomal abnormality, so further tests will be ordered.

Can ultrasound diagnose chromosomal abnormalities?

Ultrasound can sometimes increase the index of suspicion that there may be a chromosomal abnormality, but the only way to definitely diagnose whether or not one exists is to perform a more invasive test such as amniocentesis.

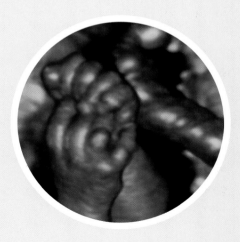

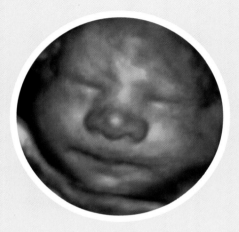

Can I get a copy of the scan?

Most hospitals will give you a copy of the scan or will allow you to purchase pictures of your baby. Usually these are printed on thermal paper, which is heat sensitive. Do not, therefore, laminate them, because this will destroy the image. To keep them forever, photocopy them or scan them into your computer.

I've heard that "walk-in" 3-D scans are available. Do you recommend them?

A lot of the information that can be gained from ultrasound scanning depends on the skill and knowledge of the sonographer. In my opinion, 3-D and 4-D ultrasound scans always must be part of a professional ultrasound examination, which includes 2-D scanning and a Doppler.

Is the baby lonely in there?

This is a question a lot of fathers ask and is an understandable reaction to the first glimpse of your baby in his own little world. But your baby probably will never again be quite so contented, warm, and comfortable once he is born. Bear in mind that an unborn baby is intimately attached to his mother and her bodily environment. This is why you should talk soothingly and reassuringly to your unborn baby and provide a stress-free, healthy environment in which to grow.

Finally, a question many dads put to me is "Don't all fetuses look alike?"

I hope the scans in this book will provide the answer!

Professor Stuart Campbell would like to thank Dr. Gonzalo Moscoso for his advice on the text and his colleages at Create Health: Dr. Geeta Nargund, Dr. Vernod Nargund, Vera Medic, and Kirsty Phillips. He'd also like to thank all the mothers who cooperated with the making of this book and who granted permission to show the scans of their babies.

All the images in *Watch Me Grow!* were taken in the Create Health Clinic, London. The majority of the images were captured by a GE Kretz Voluson 730 scanner made by General Electric; the rest of the images were taken with the Medison Accuvix.

Carroll & Brown would like to thank Sandra Schneider in bringing Professor Campbell's work to our attention.

Source of Quotations:
Page 27, Alfred, Lord Tennyson *Maud*
Page 42, Roy Dunnachie Campbell, *Home Thoughts in Bloomsbury*
Page 51, William Shakespeare, *A Midsummer Night's Dream*
Page 68, John Keats, *Letter to Benjamin Bailey, 22 November 1817*
Page 74, John Keats, *Ode to a Nightingale*
Page 83, William Wordsworth, *Nutting*
Page 88, The Bible, Proverbs
Page 94, Wilfrid Wilson Gibson, *Lament*
Page 98, Hartley Coleridge, *She is Not Fair*